VENERATING THE ROOT, PART TWO

VENERATING THE ROOT

PART TWO

Sūn Sīmiǎo

Bèi Jí Qiān Jīn Yào Fāng

(Essential Prescriptions Worth a Thousand in
Gold for Every Emergency)

孫思邈

備急千金要方

VOLUME 5: PEDIATRICS

卷五 : 少小嬰孺方

Translated by Sabine Wilms, PhD

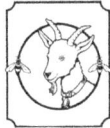

HAPPY GOAT PRODUCTIONS

PORTLAND

Published by Happy Goat Productions

Corbett, OR

Venerating the Root: A Translation of Sūn Sīmiǎo's Volume on Pediatrics in the *Bèi Jí Qiān Jīn Yào Fāng,* Part Two; translation and commmentary by Sabine Wilms

Printed in the United States of America

ISBN 978-0-9913429-8-3

Book design and layout by Kimberly Reed

Cover art by Sunjae Lee

*This book is dedicated to LOVE,
given and received by all parents, teachers,
doctors, and countless other beings who protect
little ones in the spirit of harmony between
Heaven and Earth.*

Contents

Foreword

Sabine Wilms has given us a masterful translation of Sun Simiao's treatise on pediatrics. As a pediatrician of these past 30 years who has been immersed in Chinese medicine, I had previously only read bits and pieces of this work and have been yearning for a solid translation. Well now we have one! What's more, by providing the Chinese text alongside the translation as well as superb footnotes that clarify some of the more multilayered Chinese terms, Sabine have given us a treasure that greatly expands the experience of studying the text.

In Part 1, we are given Master Sun's appreciation for the subtle developmental changes month by month that are taking place in the infant along with the management of the newborn. Throughout, he demonstrates the importance of balanced digestion and elimination in the maintenance of health and prevention of disease during childhood. We also see Sun Simiao's unique view of how possessions manifest in children. In part 2 we are given Master Sun's particular understanding of the importance of the Shanghanlun Cold School's influence during the Tang dynasty. Here we are given detailed instructions on preparing a wealth of herbal formulas for various conditions of cold damage and febrile illness from acute tidal heat to deep-lying chronic heat in children that contrasts dramatically with the one-size-fits-all approach of Tylenol that Western medicine subscribes to. While many formulas may seem antiquated, there is much to learn from how a master like Sun Simiao tweaks his formulas to respect the subtlety and tenderness of children.

At each turning of the page, we get a glimpse of the kind of medical problems Sun Simiao was called on to treat. As a seasoned pediatrician, I recognize all the common conditions we see in our practice, from caring for the newborn, to managing infantile vomiting, seizures, seasonal diarrhea, and fever. It is clear to me that Master Sun's observations could only have come from extensive clinical experience working with children. So many medical texts (both western and eastern) are steeped in heavenly theory but lack the earthy pragmatics that clinicians need in everyday practice. Unless one has been in a delivery room with a blue gasping newborn or in an emergency room with a seizing child, one may not fully appreciate the power of Master Sun's perceptions. His "pearls" of pediatrics will be of value to anyone practicing Chinese medicine who is interested in working with children. This book gives me great solace in the holistic work I am doing with children and shows me that the path I have taken over these many years venerates the root of a long and noble tradition.

Deep bows,
Stephen Scott Cowan, MD
(Happy Goat Year!)

Sun Simiao's texts are gems from a historical point of view. It is thrilling to see how advanced he was in putting down his ideas almost 1500 years ago, understanding the importance of treating children at a time when children were not as precious as they are these days. Today we have special hospitals with many wards for all kind of pediatric illnesses and we spend significant time and resources to take care of our children, pamper them, and keep them away of from any harm. However, in the old world, his approach for treating women and children first out of moral and practical reasons was considered revolutionary as he saw that treating children will create a healthier society.

Interesting to note that it took the Western world another 1000 years to write the first book about pediatric care.

But what is the importance of his writings from a clinical point of view in a world that has such strong "tools" like antibiotics and paracetamol and where vaccinations are considered compulsory in order to prevent those disease that ruled the world 1500 years ago? And on the other hand, what can we learn from the medical Gentlemen (as he beautifully calls them) who used substances that today are perceived as toxics?

Well, first of all we see that when they had to deal with life-threatening situations without the strong drugs that we have today, it made them think and search for causes for the disease so that they could eliminate and prevent them. In order to do so they were not afraid to use materials and methods that were sometimes as dangerous as the disease itself. Today we use "safer" drugs that are more potent but make us "sloppy" and therefore we may miss what is really going on in the body and what the causes for the illness are. Modern pediatric care is considered safer but is it healthier? Indeed one cannot ignore that children's mortality rate is without any doubt better than it was 1500 years ago, but does it make our children healthier ? Reading these texts about "transformations and steamings," for example, we see that in a less "comfortable" world children had different ways and reasons for being ill. This should make us wonder what is buried underneath the drugs and vaccinations we use today.

The second interesting observation relates to the fact that Chinese medicine is used today as a last line of treatment. Today we use Chinese medicine as a more gentle way to deal with or treat situations that are considered outside the focus of biomedical medicine or when parents have had enough of the symptomatic treatment of antibiotics and Tylenol. Sun Simiao's text was written in times when Chinese medicine was used when a child's life was at risk, situations that we rarely see today in our clinic as we count on the power of biomedical medicine to save the child's life. This is why his prescriptions are very strong and sometimes even much stronger than those we will use today in our clinic. This may suggest to us the potential of a good, well-diagnosed medicine that is oriented to treat the root rather than to treat the symptoms.

The last and most fascinating thing about Sun Simiao's texts is when he mentions that these texts are there in order to teach us when to treat children and when to let them heal by themselves, when a situation is life-threatening and when it is part of their normal growth. Sun Simiao emphasizes what we know but tend to forget - that children have the power to heal themselves because their Yang is so clear and that all we, as parents and medical gentlemen and gentlewomen, need to do is to guard them and guide them in their own Dao.

I want to thank Sabine for bringing these texts to us, to help all of us who cover children's ears during thunderstorms to reveal a bit more of the great mystery of human life and the ways to nourish and cultivate a healthier life for ourselves and our society.

Assaf Mor, Lic Ac. (IATcm)
Tel Aviv, 2015.

Preface

It is with great pride and joy,-- and at the same time full recognition that no book can ever be perfect,-- that Happy Goat Productions offers you this translation of the second half of Sūn Sīmiǎo's writings on pediatrics, as recorded in volume 5 of his *Bèi Jí Qiān Jīn Yào Fāng* 備急千金要方 (Essential Prescriptions Worth a Thousand in Gold for Every Emergency, completed in 652 CE).

Rather than repeating important introductory information that I have already stated in Venerating the Root, Part One (published by Happy Goat Productions in 2013), I refer the reader to pp. xvii-xxxviii of that book for a brief historical introduction to early Chinese pediatrics, to Sūn Sīmiǎo's life and work, and to the significance of pediatrics in his thinking (also accessible in electronic format at www.happygoatproductions.com).

We have maintained the layout and design of Venerating the Root, Part One by placing the original Chinese text side-by-side with my literal English translation, supplemented by my explanatory footnotes and by clinical commentary that is set off in boxes with a grey background. For this volume, I am delighted to share with you some clinical pearls by Dr. Julian Scott, the foremost practitioner of TCM pediatrics in the West and author of Natural Medicine for Children and Herbs in the Treatment of Children, which he composed in direct response to an earlier draft of this book. Throughout the book, I have also added my own commentary where needed, especially on the classical meaning of disease terms that may either not be familiar to or understood differently by practitioners of modern TCM. Last but definitely not least, as in Part One, I have translated the full

clinical commentary on this material by the famous physician
Zhāng Lù 張璐 (1617 to ca. 1700), found in his book *Qiān Jīn
Fāng Yǎn Yì* 千金方衍義 ("Expanded Meaning of the Thousand
Gold Prescriptions"). For more information on that text, as well
as on my choice of medical terminology, critical source editions
used to create the Chinese text and base my translation on, and
other details, please consult Venerating the Root, Part One.

As a rule of thumb that applies to both volumes of Venerating the Root, the format, style, lay-out, and ultimate shape of
this translation are the result of our efforts to achieve balance
between two poles: On the one hand, the need for academic
integrity and clarity, standard of translation, and faithfulness to
the historical source, and on the other hand our desire to make
this material available to a larger audience of readers who are
actively involved in the clinical application of Chinese medicine
in contemporary practice. Bridging the gulf between academia
and clinic is never an easy task, and one that is in this case
further complicated by chasms of time and space. I consider
this literal translation of Sūn Sīmiǎo's writings only a stepping
stone in the gradual development and growth of pediatrics as
an established field of specialization for practitioners of Chinese medicine over the next few decades. Given the challenges
and complexities involved in the medical treatment of children
in our current culture, this book aims to offer inspiration and
a glimpse of the possibilities, options, and rewards for practicing classical Chinese pediatrics to seasoned practitioners,
whether of contemporary biomedicine or of Chinese medicine.
We encourage you to explore the potential of this powerful spe-
cialty of Chinese medicine further in your own clinical training and practice. We furthermore hope that others will use the
information from this book to eventually create practice-ori-
ented textbooks and classes on classical Chinese pediatrics that
offer concrete instructions for diagnosis and treatment.

It is my deep conviction that the perspectives on pediatrics
offered by Sūn Sīmiǎo in the present text are an important con-
tribution to our current approach to the medical care of children,

with profound consequences for the rest of their lives. Manifesting the ideal of "treating disease before it arises," Sūn Sīmiǎo emphasizes the importance of "venerating the root" by lavishing special care on women pre-conception, during pregnancy and birth, and postpartum and while breast-feeding, and then on children, especially in the tender beginning of their lives. This is an insight that is just as pertinent today as it was in classical China 1500 years ago. It is also a truth that makes economic sense, as insurance providers and public health advocates have learned. It is worth pondering Sūn Sīmiǎo's message especially in light of our modern lifestyle with its increasingly toxic environment, growing school and performance stress for children at younger and younger ages, and ever-shrinking access to healthy whole-body activity and play, sunshine, natural foods, the outdoors, and the rhythms of nature in general. May this book inspire each of us to work collectively and individually to restore harmony between Heaven, Earth, and Humanity, for the sake of all children.

Please note that the information in this book is designed to provide historical information on the subjects discussed. For obvious reasons, it is not meant to be used, nor should it be used, to diagnose or treat any medical condition. As with any literal translation of a classical text but in particular with the subject of pediatrics, reading this book can never prepare you for clinical practice. The tender health of newborns and young children demands extensive and specialized medical training and clinical experience. The publisher and author are not responsible for any specific health or allergy needs that may require medical supervision, and are not liable for any damages or negative consequences from any treatment, action, application or preparation, to any person reading or following the information in this book.

Sabine Wilms,
Corbett, Oregon in the Year of the Happy Goat, 2015

Acknowledgments

In the spirit of this book, I would like first to acknowledge my parents, and through them also my grandparents, who all laid the foundation for this work in body, mind, and spirit. They gave me solid physical and mental health, the necessarily excessive work ethic without which a project like this would be impossible to complete, the education and experiences in multiple languages, cultures, and ages allowing me to wrap my head around this material, and unquestioning support for my strange choice of a profession through thick and thin. There is no coincidence in the fact that out of the dozens of books I have written, translated, or edited, Venerating the Root represents a breaking point that I would have never managed to go beyond without their limitless love and trust in my ability to persevere in the service of something greater than myself. I am deeply grateful for the fact that this project has given me ever-increasing clarity on the importance of "venerating the root," with innumerable good spreading in all directions like a pebble in a still pond. Whether consciously and willingly or not, my entire family of biomedical doctors has contributed to this book in more ways than they will ever know.

In the never-ending circle of family love, I have been sustained not just by my role as a daughter, but equally by my role as a mother. My sweet daughter has served as a clear-headed midwife in the long and painful pregnancy, labor, and delivery of this book by forcing me to stop and smell the roses -- and cook dinner, milk goats, walk dogs, and do laundry. Without your interruptions, my brain would have imploded a long time ago. May we enjoy a blissful and regenerative postpartum period with lots of pistachio and salted caramel ice cream before I get started on the next project!

As with the first half of Venerating the Root, this book owes its existence to the dedication, clear vision, and aesthetic of my tireless assistant and fellow Happy Goat Kim Reed (née Gray), without whose labor of love it simply wouldn't exist. For your friendship, cheerleading, enthusiasm for classical medicine, and countless shared meals and walks and moments of new-born goat love, I will be forever grateful. While your expert involvement with the layout, cover design, and formatting of this book is invaluable, your friendship is still a greater gift.

It is a great honor to have Dr. Julian Scott's pearls of insight, based on his lifelong dedication to pediatric practice, be a part of this book. Without ever having met you in person, your kind response to Part One made a world of difference in my recognition of the clinical value of this material and gave me a much-needed boost to continue on with Part Two. Also thanks to Dr. Michael Weber, for introducing us to each other! Likewise, I am delighted to include a short preface by Dr. Stephen Cowan, an experienced pediatrician who is able to bridge the gap between modern biomedicine and Chinese medicine in his practice. Nothing makes me happier than to hear that this ancient information is proving useful in modern clinical practice. Academics are not used to receiving this kind of enthusiastic response and I never take it for granted. I am excited to see what the shared future of our medicine may look like in the hands of physicians like Dr. Cowan.

I owe mountains of gratitude to my dear friends, colleagues, and teachers at the School of Classical Chinese Medicine at the National College of Natural Medicine, most notably Drs. Brenda Hood, Ri-hui Long, Heiner Fruehauf, and Laurie Regan, and to all the other beautiful doctors who I have the great fortune to cross paths with on a regular basis. From Debra Betts in New Zealand to Assaf Mor in Israel, Michael Weber in Germany, Julian Scott in the UK, Scott Tower, Genevieve LeGoff, and Stephen Cowan in the US, I am humbled by your work and consider myself so lucky to be contributing in a small way to your practices. In your passion and deep-hearted dedication to a life of service as true healers, you demonstrate every day how powerful Sūn Sīmiǎo's vision of the "Eminent Physician" is in modern clinical practice.

Of course this list would not be complete without acknowledging the debt I owe to my students at the National College of Natural Medicine in Portland, Oregon, and the readers of my books, visitors to my website, and attendants at my lectures and seminars worldwide. Thank you for caring, for sharing my love for this material, and for asking often unanswerable questions that force me to reconsider preconceived notions I have held based on my previous training and experiences. It is due to the support and response from our beautiful community of Chinese medicine practitioners (in the largest sense of that word) that I have been able to complete yet another book of several hundred pages on a shoestring budget. I truly feel that this book is not my work at all, but the result of our collective recognition, as a profession, that Sūn Sīmiǎo's ancient words of wisdom are as relevant and important today as they were in medieval China. I thank you all for making this book possible.

Last but definitely not least, I thank all the animal mothers on my farm who have kindly allowed me to witness their mastery of the art of "nurturing the small" in action, from goats to dogs, cats, sheep, geese, turkeys, and bees. I have learned so much about the beauty of life from every one of you proud mamas.

Chapter Five - Cold Damage

傷寒第五

(1 essay, 35 formulas, 1 moxibustion method)

論曰:

（一）夫小兒未能冒涉霜雪，乃不病傷寒也。

（二）大人解脫之久，傷於寒冷，則不論耳。

（三）然天行非節之氣，其亦得之。

（四）有時行疾疫之年，小兒出腹便患斑者也，治其時行節度，故如大人法，但用藥分劑小異，藥小冷耳。

V.1 Essay[1]

(1) The reason why small children cannot yet be exposed to frost and snow is so that they do not fall ill with cold damage.

(2) Since adults have been released [from this concern] for a long time, their damage from cold is not worth talking about.

(3) Nevertheless, when heaven sends down qì that is outside of its proper season, they also contract [cold damage] from it.[2]

(4) In years with seasonal epidemics, when small children suffer from macules right when they emerge from the [mother's] abdomen,[3] treat [the condition] in accordance with the proper seasonal progression. Therefore it is like the methods for adults. The only difference is that the usage and dosage of the medicine differs slightly and that the medicines are slightly cooler.

---

1 It may be important for historically-minded readers that the following essay is not found in the *Sūn Zhēn Rén* edition, which predates the involvement of the Sòng period editorial team. So it might be an addition dating from long after Sūn Sīmiǎo's lifetime.

2 I read this line as explaining that even adults contract cold damage conditions when it is a case of unseasonal qì, while children can contract cold damage not just from unseasonal qì but even from cold that is occurring in its proper seasonal progression and hence must be protected from cold at all times. Several other editions of the *Qiān Jīn Fāng* however, lack the second line that comments on adult conditions of cold damage. In that case, line 3 has to refer to newborn children also contracting diseases that are caused by unseasonal qì, in addition to conditions that are caused simply by their being exposed to cold and not yet having sufficiently strong bodies to endure it.

3 In several editions of the *Qiān Jīn Fāng*, including the *Yǎn Yì* version, the character 便 *biàn*, which I here interpret as "right away," is replaced with 但 *dàn*, which usually means "only" or occasionally "however," but can also be used like 就 *jiù* in the sense of "then" or "right away." *Biàn* can have a similar meaning of "contrary to one's expectations," which is another way that this line could be read, since the baby is suffering from macules before ever being exposed to any external pathogens or presents with macules instead of the standard signs of seasonal epidemics.

麥門冬湯

治小兒未滿百日傷寒，鼻衄身熱嘔逆方。

麥門冬	十八銖
石膏	各半兩
寒水石	
甘草	
桂心	八銖

上五味，咬咀，以水二升半，煮取一升，分服一合，日三。

V.2 Màiméndōng Tāng (Ophiopogon Decoction)

Indication

A formula for small children less than a hundred days old, to treat cold damage with nosebleeds, generalized heat [effusion], and counterflow retching.

Ingredients

màiméndōng	18 *zhū*
shígāo	
hánshuǐshí	0.5 *liǎng* each
gāncǎo	
guìxīn	8 *zhū*

Preparation

Pound the five ingredients above and decoct in 2.5 *shēng* of water until reduced to 1 *shēng*. Divide and take in doses of 1 *gě*, three times a day.

麥門冬湯《衍義》

（一）初生小兒斑衄嘔逆，多由稟體之弱，寒邪入犯而蘊熱。

（二）與大人之伏氣發溫無異。

（三）所以專取白虎，而兼竹葉、石膏、炙甘草湯之製，以寒水石代知母而化腎熱，麥門冬代粳米而滋肺腎。

（四）其用桂心，妙義有三：

（五）一保初生陽氣，一發諸藥性味，一為散熱嚮導。

（六）即伏氣發溫時行疫病，當不出此。倘表證未除，不妨仍用桂枝，不失南陽本來聖法。

Màiméndōng Tāng (Japanese Hyacinth Tuber Decoction) *Yǎn Yì* (Expanded Meaning)

(1) When newborn babies suffer from macules, nose-bleeds, and counterflow retching, in the majority of cases this is due to a weakness in the endowed constitution, allowing cold evil to invade and cause accumulated heat.

(2) This is no different from deep-lying qì effusing as warmth in adults.

(3) For this reason, [Sūn Sīmiǎo] has specifically chosen Báihǔ Tāng and combined it with Zhúyè Tāng, Shígāo Tāng, and Zhì Gāncǎo Tāng for this preparation. [The present formula] substitutes *hánshuǐshí* for *zhīmǔ*, to transform the heat in the kidney, and *màiméndōng* for *jīngmǐ*, to enrich the lung and kidney.

(4) Its use of *guìxīn* is ingenious in three ways:

(5) First, it safeguards the newborn's yáng qì. Second, it brings out the special characteristics and flavors of the various other medicinals. And third, it functions to disperse heat and guide it [out].

(6) In cases of deep-lying qì effusing as warmth in seasonal epidemics, you should not go beyond [these medicinals either]. In the event that the exterior pattern is not yet eliminated, you can still use *guìzhī* with no harm. Thus you do not lose the sage's method that originally came [from Zhāng Zhòngjǐng] from Nányáng.

芍藥四物解肌湯

治少小傷寒方。

芍藥	
黃芩	各半兩
升麻	
葛根	

（一）上四味，㕮咀，以水三升，煮取九合，去
滓，分服。

（二）期歲以上分三服。

芍藥四物解肌湯《衍義》

（一）此升麻湯兼黃芩湯之製。

（二）以升麻湯專行陽明，黃芩湯專走少陽，此
則兼解二經風熱也。

V.3 Sháoyào Sì Wù Jiě Jī Tāng (Peony Four-Ingredient Flesh-Resolving Decoction)

Indication
A formula to treat cold damage in childhood.

Ingredients

sháoyào	
huángqín	0.5 *liǎng* each
shēngmá	
gégēn	

Preparation
(1) Pound the four ingredients above and decoct in 3 *shēng* of water until reduced to 9 *gě*. Remove the dregs and divide into doses.

(2) For an infant older than a full year, divide into three doses.

> ### Sháoyào Sì Wù Jiě Jī Tāng (Peony Four-Ingredient Flesh-Resolving Decoction) *Yǎn Yì* (Expanded Meaning)
>
> (1) This [formula] is a preparation that combines Shēngmá Tāng and Huángqín Tāng.
>
> (2) It uses Shēngmá Tāng to specifically go to the Yángmíng [level], and Huángqín Tāng to specifically address the Shàoyáng [level]. In this way, the present formula resolves wind heat in both of these channels.

麻黃湯

治少小傷寒，發熱咳嗽頭面熱者方。

麻黃	
生薑	各一兩
黃芩	
甘草	
石膏	各半兩
芍藥	
杏仁	十枚
桂心	半兩

（一）上八味，咬咀，以水四升，煮取一升半，
　　　分二服。

（二）兒若小，以意減之。

V.4 Máhuáng Tāng (Ephedra Decoction)

Indication

A formula for children, to treat cold damage that presents with fever, coughing, and heat in the head and face.

Ingredients

máhuáng	1 *liǎng* each
shēngjiāng	
huángqín	
gāncǎo	0.5 *liǎng* each
shígāo	
sháoyào	
xìngrén	ten pieces
guìxīn	0.5 *liǎng*

Preparation

(1) Pound the eight ingredients above and decoct in 4 *shēng* of water until reduced to 1.5 *shēng*. Divide into two doses.

(2) If the child is still small, reduce [the dosage] at your discretion.

麻黃湯《衍義》

（一）此本南陽先師麻黃湯、麻杏石甘湯，兼越
　　　脾湯、桂枝麻黃各半湯等方之製。

（二）其間但不用大棗者，以嬰兒臟腑窄弱，恐
　　　其戀膈助滿也。

（三）與前芍藥四物解肌湯不用甘草同義。

（四）此有桂心辛散，則甘草又為必需。

Máhuáng Tāng (Ephedra Decoction) *Yǎn Yì* (Expanded Meaning)

(1) This is a preparation that combines the original formulas for Máhuáng Tāng and Má Xìng Shí Gān Tāng by the Esteemed Master [Zhāng Zhòngjǐng] from Nányáng with Yuèpí Tāng and Guìzhī Máhuáng Gè Bàn Tāng.

(2) The only ingredient that [the present formula] does not include is *dàzǎo*. The reason for this is that the *zàng* and *fǔ* organs are constricted and weak in infants, and I fear that [its tendency] to adhere to the diaphragm might assist the [pathological] fullness.

(3) It is for this same reason that *gāncǎo* was omitted from the previous formula for Sháoyào Sì Wù Jiě Jī Tāng.

(4) The present formula [however] contains *guìxīn*, which is acrid and dissipating. For this reason, *gāncǎo* is here a necessity.

葛根汁

治小兒傷寒方。

葛根汁	各六合
淡竹瀝	

（一）上二味相和。

（二）二三歲兒分三服，百日兒斟酌服之。

（三）不宜生，煮服佳。

葛根汁《衍義》

（一）葛根搗汁，以散陽明客邪，淡竹炙瀝，以
　　　清胃中痰熱。

（二）不宜生服者，恐其寒滑作瀉也。

V.5 Gégēn Zhī (Pueraria Juice)

Indication
A formula to treat cold damage in small children.

Ingredients

gégēnzhī	6 *gě* each
dànzhúlì	

Preparation
(1) Mix the two ingredients above together.

(2) For a child aged two to three *suì*, divide into three doses. For a child within the first hundred days of life, dose it according to your deliberations.

(3) It is not appropriate to give [this juice] raw. Boiling it first before you have [the patient] ingest it is best.

Gégēn Zhī (Pueraria Juice) *Yǎn Yì* (Expanded Meaning)

(1) The juice from pounded *gégēn* is used to dissipate intrusive evil in the Yángmíng level. The sap from roasted *dànzhú* is used to clear phlegm heat from inside the stomach.

(2) The reason for the prohibition against taking [this juice] raw is that I fear that the cold and slippery [nature of the raw ingredients] will cause diarrhea.

小兒時氣方

（一）桃葉三兩搗，以水五升，煮十沸取汁。

（二）日五六遍淋之。

（三）若複發，燒雄鼠屎二枚，燒水調服之。

《衍義》

（一）桃葉專闢一切時行不正之氣。

（二）若淋之蒸之，其熱不解，此必素稟腎虛，
　　　邪乘於里。

（三）故燒猳鼠屎以祛內陷之熱也。

V.6 Formula for Seasonal Qì in Small Children

(1) Pound 3 *liǎng* of peach leaves and decoct in 5 *shēng* of water, bringing it to a boil ten times. Take the liquid.

(2) Drizzle this on the patient five to six times a day.

(3) If [the condition] erupts again, char two pieces of male mouse droppings and [have the patient] ingest them mixed into heated water.

Yǎn Yì (Expanded Meaning)

(1) Peach leaves specifically repel all seasonal qì that is not right.

(2) If the patient's heat still fails to resolve after you have treated them by drizzling [the decoction] on them or exposing them to the steam, this must [mean] a constitutional inherited kidney vacuity that is allowing the evil to overwhelm the interior.

(3) This is the reason why charred boar or mice droppings are [then] used to dispel the internally trapped heat.

五味子湯

治小兒傷寒，病久不除，瘥後複劇，瘦瘠骨立方。

五味子	十銖
甘草	各十二銖
當歸	
大黃	六銖
芒硝	五銖
麥門冬	各六銖
黃芩	
前胡	
石膏	一兩
黃連	六銖

（一）上十味，咬咀，以水三升，煮取一升半，服二合。

（二）得下便止，計大小增減之。

V.7 Wǔwèizǐ Tāng (Schisandra Decoction)

Indication

A formula that treats cold damage in small children, when the disease has become chronic and cannot be eliminated but returns with a vengeance after each recovery, [resulting in] emaciation and frailty to the point of showing the bones.

Ingredients

wǔwèizǐ	10 *zhū*
gāncǎo	12 *zhū* each
dāngguī	
dàhuáng	6 *zhū*
mángxiāo	5 *zhū*
màiméndōng	6 *zhū* each
huángqín	
qiánhú	
shígāo	1 *liǎng*
huánglián	6 *zhū*

Preparation

(1) Pound the ten ingredients above and decoct in 3 *shēng* of water until reduced to 1.5 *shēng*. Take in doses of 2 *gě* each.

(2) Stop as soon as you have induced a downward movement.[4] Increase or decrease the dosage in accordance with the patient's size.

---

4   得下: I have translated this phrase literally, but here it clearly refers to the medicine's action of inducing a bowel movement, which indicates the elimination of the pathogenic agent in the stool. In medical literature, the action of a formula or medicinal that is described as 下 includes moving the pathogenic factor not just down but also out, or in other words, elimination via urine and/or stool.

五味子湯《衍義》

（一）小兒傷寒，病久不除，或瘥後復劇，此必邪從火化而陷伏不解，所以瘦瘠骨立。

（二）非急投三黃下奪，無以洩之，三黃不逮，濟以芒硝，石膏。

（三）其前胡、麥冬、五味、甘草、當歸以滋津氣之燥。

（四）在嬰兒固為合劑，以元神未動，不慮其引邪納賊也。

Wǔwèizǐ Tāng (Schisandra Decoction) *Yǎn Yì* (Expanded Meaning)

(1) When cold damage in small children becomes chronic and cannot be eliminated or returns with a vengeance after the patient has recovered, this must mean that evil has transmuted from fire and become trapped deep inside instead of resolving. This is the reason for the emaciation and frailty to the point of showing the bones.

(2) If you do not quickly give the patient the "three *huáng*"[5] to "wrestle" [the disease] down and out, you will have no other way of discharging it. And for whatever the three *huáng* fail to capture, rescue [the patient] with *mángxiāo* and *shígāo*.

(3) The *qiánhú, màiméndōng, wǔwèizǐ, gāncǎo,* and *dāngguī* in this formula are used to irrigate the dryness of the liquids and qì.

(4) For infants, [this formula] functions securely as a combination preparation, so that you don't have to worry about attracting evil and allowing in thieves [at a time] when the source spirit is not active yet.[6]

---

5   三黄: Literally, "three yellows," here this term is an abbreviation for the three medicinals of the formula that contain the character 黄 in their names: *dàhuáng, huángqín,* and *huánglián.*

6   The exact meaning of the expression 元神未動 "the source spirit is not active yet" is unclear to me. It hinges on our understanding of the function of the "source spirit" in newborn children, and the significance of its movement or activity, whether physiological or pathological. To further complicate matters, this phrase is found in the commentary, which dates from the seventeenth century, rather than in the original text. It is therefore important to contemplate the understanding of 元神 *yuán shén* during that period in addition to its conceptualization by Sūn Sīmiǎo and his contemporaries. It is also possible that the movement (動) refers to pathological stirring as opposed to healthy activity. My best guess, based on context, is that the lack or weakness of physiological activity by the source spirit might be related to the baby's ability to defend her- or himself against external evils.

浴湯

莽草湯

治少小傷寒浴方。

莽草	半斤
牡蠣	四兩
雷丸	三十枚
蛇床子	一升
大黃	一兩

（一）上五味，㕮咀，以水三斗，煮取一斗半。

（二）適寒溫以浴兒，避眼及陰。

V.8 Wash Decoctions

V.8.a Mǎngcǎo Tāng (Japanese Star Anise Decoction)[7], Version One

Indication
A formula for a wash to treat cold damage in children.

Ingredients

mǎngcǎo	0.5 *jīn*
mǔlì	4 *liǎng*
léiwán	30 pieces
shéchuángzǐ	1 *shēng*
dàhuáng	1 *liǎng*

Preparation
(1) Pound the five ingredients above and decoct in 3 *dǒu* of water until reduced to 1.5 *dǒu*.

(2) Adjust the temperature and use the decoction to wash the child with. Avoid the eyes and genitals.

---

7 *Mǎngcǎo* is a highly toxic substance traditionally used to catch fish by poisoning them so that they float to the surface, and in medicine as a fumigant or ingredient in washing decoctions. This plant is related but not identical to (Chinese) star anise, which is used as a spice.

莽草湯

治小兒猝寒熱，不佳，不能服藥方浴方。

莽草	各三兩
丹參	
桂心	
菖蒲	半斤
蛇床子	一兩
雷丸	一升

（一）上六味，咬咀，以水二斗，煮三五沸。

（二）適寒溫以浴兒，避眼及陰。

V.8.b Măngcǎo Tāng (Japanese Star Anise Decoction)[8], Version Two

Indication

A formula for a wash to treat small children with unexpected attacks of [aversion to] cold and heat [effusion] and unwellness, who are unable to take medicine internally.

Ingredients

măngcǎo	
dānshēn	3 *liǎng* each
guìxīn	
chāngpú	0.5 *jīn*
shéchuángzǐ	1 *liǎng*
léiwán	1 *shēng*

Preparation

(1) Pound the six ingredients above and decoct in 2 *dǒu* of water, bringing it to a boil fifteen times.

(2) Adjust the temperature until it is comfortable and wash the child with this. Avoid the eyes and genitals.

---

8   This formula does in fact carry the same name as the previous formula.

雷丸湯

治小兒忽寒熱浴方。

雷丸	二十枚
大黃	四兩
苦參	三兩
黃芩	一兩
丹參	二兩
石膏	三兩

（一）上六味，咬咀，以水二斗，煮取一斗半。

（二）浴兒，避眼及陰。

（三）浴訖，以粉粉之，勿濃衣，一宿複浴。

李葉湯

治少小身熱浴方。

李葉無多少，咬咀，以水煮，去滓，將浴兒良。

V.8.c Léiwán Tāng (Omphalia Decoction)

Indication

A formula for a wash to treat small children with sudden [aversion to] cold and heat [effusion].

Ingredients

léiwán	20 pieces
dàhuáng	4 *liǎng*
kǔshēn	3 *liǎng*
huángqín	1 *liǎng*
dānshēn	2 *liǎng*
shígāo	3 *liǎng*

Preparation

(1) Pound the six ingredients above and decoct in 2 *dǒu* of water until reduced to 1.5 *dǒu*.

(2) Wash the child with this, avoiding the eyes and genitals.

(3) When you are finished with the wash, sprinkle powder on them. Do not dress them too warmly and repeat this wash treatment after one night.

V.8.d Plum Leaf Decoction

Indication

A formula for a wash to treat generalized heat in children.

Ingredients and Preparation

Pound an unspecified amount of plum leaves, decoct in water, and remove the dregs. Using this to wash the child is excellent.

柳枝湯

治小兒生一月至五月，乍寒乍熱方。

（一）細切柳枝，煮取汁，洗兒。

（二）若渴，絞冬瓜汁服之。

V.8.e Willow Twig Decoction

Indication

A formula to treat small children who are suffering from rapidly fluctuating cold and heat in the first one to five months of their life.

Ingredients and Preparation

(1) Finely chop willow twigs, and decoct them. Take the juice and wash the child with this.

(2) If [the patient is also suffering from] thirst, sqeeze *dōngguā* to get the juice and [have the patient] ingest that.

青木香湯

治小兒壯熱羸瘠方。

青木香	四兩
麻子仁	一升
虎骨	五兩
白芷	三兩
竹葉	一升

上五味，咬咀，以水二斗，煮取一斗，稍稍浴兒。

《衍義》

（一）已上六方，皆取其盪邪熱，逐毒氣之功。

（二）宜諒稟質隨時取用。

V.8.f Qīngmùxiāng Tāng (Aristolochia Decoction)

Indication
A formula to treat small children suffering from serious fever and emaciation and frailty.

Ingredients

qīngmùxiāng	4 *liǎng*
mázǐrén	1 *shēng*
hǔgǔ	5 *liǎng*
báizhǐ	3 *liǎng*
zhúyè	1 *shēng*

Preparation
Pound the five ingredients above and decoct in 2 *dǒu* of water until reduced to 1 *dǒu*. Little by little, wash the child with this.

Yǎn Yì (Expanded Meaning)

(1) All the six formulas above have the intended effect of flushing out evil heat and expelling toxic qì.

(2) It is advised to take [the patient's] endowed constitution into consideration whenever you choose to use them.

李根湯

治小兒暴有熱，得之二三日方。

李根	
桂心	各十八銖
芒硝	
甘草	各一兩
麥門冬	

上五味，咬咀，以水三升，煮取一升，分五服。

李根湯《衍義》

（一）李根咸寒降火，芒消苦寒蕩熱，麥冬、甘草甘平滋津，桂心辛溫破結。

（二）熱因熱用，從治之法也。

V.9 Lǐgēn Tāng (Plum Root Decoction)

Indication

A formula to treat fulminant presence of heat in small children, [to use] two or three days after they contracted it.

Ingredients

lǐgēn	18 *zhū* each
guìxīn	
mángxiāo	
gāncǎo	1 *liǎng* each
màiméndōng	

Preparation

Pound the five ingredients above and decoct in 3 *shēng* of water until reduced to 1 *shēng*. Divide into five doses.

Lǐgēn Tāng (Plum Root Decoction) *Yǎn Yì* (Expanded Meaning)

(1) *Lǐgēn* is salty and cold and causes fire to descend. *Mángxiāo* is bitter and cold and flushes out heat. *Màiméndōng* and *gāncǎo* are sweet and neutral and enrich the fluids. *Guìxīn* is acrid and warm and breaks up binds.

(2) Using heat to treat heat, [this formula] is based on the method of "conforming treatment."[9]

---

9 從治 *cóng zhì*: Literally "following treatment," Wiseman translates this as "coacting treatment." Also known as 反治 *fǎn zhì* ("paradoxical treatment"), this method describes the apparently paradoxical therapeutic principle of treating signs of a certain pathology with medicinals that induce that very action. In the present case, for example, signs of heat are treated with heat-inducing medicinals. This approach only makes sense once you recognize that the signs of heat here are misleading and do in fact indicate an underlying pathology of the opposite nature, namely an exuberance of cold on the inside that is forcing vacuous yáng to stray to the surface, where it manifests in signs of false heat.

十二物寒水石散

治少小身體壯熱，不能服藥粉方。

寒水石
芒硝
滑石
石膏
赤石脂
青木香
大黃
甘草
黃芩
防風
芎藭
麻黃根

上各等分，合治下篩，以粉一升，藥屑三合相
和，複以篩篩之，以粉兒身，日三。

V.10 Shíèr Wù Hánshuǐshí Sǎn (Twelve-Ingredient Glauberite Powder)

Indication

To treat severe generalized heat in children, a formula for a powder, when the child is unable to take medicine internally.

Ingredients

hánshuǐshí
mángxiāo
huáishí
shígāo
chìshízhī
qīngmùxiāng
dàhuáng
gāncǎo
huángqín
fángfēng
xiōngqióng
máhuánggēn

Preparation

Combine equal amounts of the ingredients above and finely pestle and sift them. Take 1 *shēng* of rice flour and combine with 3 *gě* of the ground-up medicine. Sift it one more time with a sieve. Sprinkle this powder on the child's body three times a day.

十二物寒水石散《衍義》

（一）一派苦寒闢熱藥中，只取防風一味達表。

（二）石膏一味實裡，麻黃根一味斂汗，尤賴米
　　　粉以實肌肉。

Shíèr Wù Hánshuǐshí Sǎn (Twelve-Ingredient Glauberite Powder) *Yǎn Yì* (Expanded Meaning)

(1) From the whole group of bitter and cold medicinals that repel heat, [this formula] uses only the single ingredient *fángfēng* to outthrust the exterior.

(2) With *shígāo* as the only ingredient to make the interior replete, and *máhuánggēn* as the only ingredient to restrain sweating, this formula relies particularly on rice flour to make the flesh replete.

升麻湯

治小兒傷寒，變熱毒病，身熱面赤，口燥，心腹堅急，大小便不利，或口瘡者，或因壯熱，便四肢攣掣驚，仍成癇疾，時發時醒，醒後身熱如火者，悉主之方。

升麻	
白薇	
麻黃	
葳蕤	各半兩
柴胡	
甘草	
黃芩	一兩
朴硝	
大黃	各六銖
鉤藤	

V.11 Shēngmá Tāng (Cimicifuga Decoction)

Indication

A formula for small children, to treat cold damage that has transformed into a disease of heat toxin, with generalized heat and a red face, dry mouth, hardness and tension in the heart and abdomen, inhibited defecation and urination, possibly with sores in the mouth, or with serious heat that is causing spasms in the four limbs, tugging, and fright,[10] then developing into [full-blown] seizures with intermittent outbreaks and [periods of] consciousness, with generalized heat that is like fire after the person regains consciousness. This formula treats it all.

Ingredients

shēngmá	
báiwēi	
máhuáng	0.5 *liǎng* each
wěiruí	
cháihú	
gāncǎo	
huángqí	1 *liǎng*
pòxiāo	
dàhuáng	6 *zhū* each
gōuténg	

---

10 For more on the concept of "fright" (驚 *jīng*), see *Venerating the Root, Part One*, especially Chapter Three on "Fright Seizures." It is important to keep in mind that the concept in the technical medical sense does not refer so much to the actual experience of being exposed to something frightening but rather to a specific intense physical response of being thrown into a state of panic or shock. As the horse radical 馬 in this character suggests, the best way to understand "fright" is perhaps to visualize a horse that is rearing up in panic. In the context of neonatal physiology, the key characteristic of this symptom is the explosive and extremely dangerous scattering of qì in a counterflow upward direction, which is the precise opposite of the healthy physiological consolidation, gathering in, and "grounding" in its manifestation on Earth that is so essential during the first few months of a newborn's life.

（一）上十味，咬咀，以水三升，先煮麻黄，去上沫，納諸藥，煮取一升。

（二）兒生三十日至六十日，一服二合； 六十日至百日，一服二合半； 百日至二百日，一服三合。

升麻湯《衍義》

（一）此採麻黄升麻湯中五味，以二麻透表，黄芩洩熱，蔞、甘潤燥。

（二）參入白薇散堅，柴胡退熱，硝、黄蕩實，鈎藤舒攣。

（三）表裡兼治之捷法，仍從南陽法中化出。

Preparation

(1) Pound the ten ingredients above. First decoct the *máhuáng* in 3 *shēng* of water and remove the foam from the top. Add the other medicinals and decoct until reduced to 1 *shēng*.

(2) For a child within the first thirty to sixty days after birth, one dose is 2 *gě*. Between sixty and a hundred days after birth, one dose is 2.5 *gě*. Between a hundred and two hundred days after birth, one dose is 3 *gě*.

Shēngmá Tāng (Cimicifuga Decoction) *Yǎn Yì* (Expanded Meaning)

(1) This formula has picked five ingredients from the formula for Máhuáng Shēngmá Tāng[11]: the "two *má*"[12] to outthrust the exterior, *huángqín* to discharge heat, and *wěiruí* and *gāncǎo* to moisten dryness.

(2) [These medicinals] are joined by *báiwēi* to disperse hardness, *cháihú* to abate heat, *pòxiāo* and *dàhuáng* to flush out repletion, and *gōuténg* to soothe spasms.

(3) This nimble method for treating the interior and exterior simultaneously is still derived from a transformation of the method [of Zhāng Zhòngjǐng] from Nányáng.

---

11 This formula from the *Shāng Hán Lùn* is indicated there for the following condition: "On the sixth or seventh day of cold damage, after major downward movement, [if you see] a sunken and slow *cùn* pulse, reversal counterflow in the hands and feet, failure of the pulse to reach the lower part of the body, inhibition in the throat, and vomiting of pus and blood."

12 二麻 *èr má*: *shēngmá* and *máhuáng*.

大黃湯

治小兒肉中挾宿熱，瘦瘠，熱進退休作無時方。

大黃	各半兩
甘草	
芒硝	
桂心	八銖
石膏	一兩
大棗	五枚

上六味，咬咀，以水三升，煮取一升，每服二合。

V.12 Formulas for Dàhuáng Tāng (Rhubarb Decoctions)

V.12.a Dàhuáng Tāng (Rhubarb Decoction)

Indication

A formula for small children that treats conditions of heat chronically abiding inside the flesh, [manifesting] with emaciation and frailty and with the heat advancing and abating, being active and at rest with no regularity.

Ingredients

dàhuáng	0.5 *liǎng* each
gāncǎo	
mángxiāo	
guìxīn	8 *zhū*
shígāo	1 *liǎng*
dàzǎo	5 pieces

Preparation

Pound the six ingredients above and decoct in 3 *shēng* of water until reduced to 1 *shēng*. Take 2 *gě* per dose.

治小兒腹大短氣，熱有進退，食不安，穀為不化方。

大黃	各半兩
黃芩	
甘草	
芒硝	
麥門冬	
石膏	一兩
桂心	八銖

（一）上七味，咬咀，以水三升，煮取一升半，分三服。

（二）期歲以下兒作五服。

V.12.b Another Formula[13]

Indication

A formula for small children to treat an enlarged abdomen and shortness of breath, with heat that advances and abates, unease when eating, and failure to transform grain.

Ingredients

dàhuáng	
huángqín	
gāncǎo	0.5 *liǎng* each
mángxiāo	
màiméndōng	
shígāo	1 *liǎng*
guìxīn	8 *zhū*

Preparation

(1) Pound the seven ingredients above and decoct in 3 *shēng* of water until reduced to 1.5 *shēng*. Divide into three doses.

(2) For a child younger than one year, divide into five doses.

---

13 In the present edition, I have moved this formula up from its position in standard received versions of the *Qiān Jīn Fāng*, where it is found below the following formula for Shǔqī Sǎn. The reason for my decision is that the *Yǎn Yì* edition contains an explanation that applies to both versions of Dàhuáng Tāng and that it is helpful to look at them side by side. Given the fact that the order and location of formulas is by no means fixed between different older manuscript editions of the *Qiān Jīn Fāng* but even varies between different chapters, it is impossible at this point to restore the original order of formulas with certainty. For this reason, I have taken the liberty of following the *Yǎn Yì* edition here

大黃湯《衍義》

（一）前方以肉中久挾宿熱，故用大棗引硝、黃、甘、石入於營分，然非桂心，無以散之。

（二）後方以腹大短氣，故用黃芩、麥冬，引硝、黃、甘、石入於氣分，仍用桂心為嚮導耳。

Dàhuáng Tāng (Rhubarb Decoctions) *Yǎn Yì* (Expanded Meaning)

(1) Because the first formula above addresses chronically abiding heat in the flesh, it uses *dàzǎo* to pull *mángxiāo*, *dàhuáng*, *gāncǎo*, and *shígāo* into the *yíng* provisioning level. Nevertheless, if [the formula] didn't include *guìxīn*, it would not be able to dissipate [the heat].

(2) The second formula above addresses an enlarged abdomen and shortness of breath and therefore uses *huángqín* and *màiméndōng* to pull *mángxiāo*, *dàhuáng*, *gāncǎo*, and *shígāo* into the qì level. [Like the previous formula], it still uses *guìxīn* to lead the way.

蜀漆湯

治小兒潮熱方。

蜀漆	
甘草	
知母	各半兩
龍骨	
牡蠣	

（一）上五味，咬咀，以水四升，煮取一升，去滓。

（二）一歲兒少少溫服半合，日再。

V.13 Shǔqī Tāng (Dichroa Leaf Decoction)

Indication
A formula for tidal heat in small children.

Ingredients

shǔqī	
gāncǎo	
zhīmǔ	0.5 liǎng each
lónggǔ	
mǔlì	

Preparation
(1) Pound the five ingredients above and decoct in 4 shēng of water until reduced to 1 shēng. Remove the dregs.

(2) For a child within the first year of life, give a little at a time, warm, in doses of 0.5 gě twice a day.

蜀漆湯《衍義》

（一）此即《金匱》蜀漆散，彼治大人牡瘧，故
用漿水欵蜀漆以搜痰涎。

（二）此治小兒潮熱，故用知母佐牡蠣以靜伏
熱。

（三）用甘草者即《外台》牡蠣湯，去麻黄而易
知母，一從表散，一從內解，兩不移易之
定法。

Shǔqī Tāng (Dichroa Leaf Decoction) *Yǎn Yì* (Expanded Meaning)

(1) This formula is identical with [the formula for] Shǔqī Sǎn from the *Jīn Guì Yào Lüè*. That formula treats male malaria in adults and hence uses *jiāngshuǐ* to detain the *shǔqī*, in order to rout the phlegm and drool.[14]

(2) The present formula treats tidal heat in small children and therefore uses *zhīmǔ* to assist the *mǔlì* in quieting the deep-lying heat.

(3) Its use of *gāncǎo* here is identical with [the rationale behind] Mǔlì Tāng in the *Wài Tái Mì Yào*, except that it has removed *máhuáng* and replaced it with *zhīmǔ*. While one formula dissipates from the exterior, the other resolves from the interior. Neither of them alter the fixed method of [treating by] transformation.

---

14 The *Yǎn Yì* text here contains numerous mistakes, which, when read literally, make it incomprehensible. First, the character 涏 *tǐng* needs to be changed to 涎 *xián*, meaning "drool." Second, and more importantly, the punctuation of the modern editors (as 故用漿水、款、蜀漆以搜痰涎。) is misleading and based on an erroneous understanding of the original source, which did not contain punctuation marks. The meaning with that punctuation would be "Therefore it uses *jiāngshuǐ, kuǎndōnghuā*, and *shǔqī* to track down phlegm and drool." The original formula for Shǔqī Sǎn from the *Jīn Guì Yào Lüè*, however, does not contain *kuǎndōnghuā* but merely *shǔqī, yúnmǔ,* and *lónggǔ*, in equal amounts. These medicinals are to be ingested mixed with *jiāngshuǐ* before the onset of a malaria episode. The character 款 *kuǎn* therefore does not refer to a medicinal ingredient here but needs to be read in its historical meaning as "detaining," in the sense of entertaining guests and thereby making them stay. This meaning, while rare, fits beautifully with the intention of the formula.

竹葉湯

治小兒夏月患腹中伏熱，溫壯來往，或患下痢，色或白或黃，三焦不利竹葉湯方。

竹葉	切，五合
小麥	三合
柴胡	半兩
黃芩	一兩六銖
茯苓	十八銖
人參	各半兩
麥門冬	
甘草	

V.14 Formulas for Vigorous Warmth

V.14.a Zhúyè Tāng (Bamboo Leaf Decoction), Version One

Indication

A formula for small children who are suffering from deep lying heat inside the abdomen during the summer months, with intermittently occurring vigorous warmth,[15] possibly suffering from diarrhea as well that is either whitish or yellowish in color, with inhibition in the triple burner.

Ingredients

zhúyè	chopped, 5 *gě*
xiǎomài	3 *gě*
cháihú	0.5 *liǎng*
huángqín	1 *liǎng*, 6 *zhū*
fúlíng	18 *zhū*
rénshēn	0.5 *liǎng* each
màiméndōng	
gāncǎo	

---

15 溫壯: *wēn zhuàng* ("vigorous warmth") is a technical term describing a febrile condition in small children. In the *Zhū Bìng Yuán Hòu Lùn*, it is explained as "caused by disharmony in the *zàng* and *fǔ* organs, the presence of deep-lying heat, or abiding cold, all of which have spread to [affect] stomach qì. The Foot Yángmíng Stomach Channel governs the flesh in the body, and when a person's stomach is not harmonious, the movement of qì becomes congested so that [the qì] smolders and gathers, causing heat in the body. The symptom in small children is as follows: If the feces are yellow and foul-smelling, this means deep-lying heat inside the abdomen, which should be treated with Lóngdǎn Tāng. If the feces are white and sour-smelling, this means abiding cold failing to disperse, which should be treated with Zǐ Shuāng Wán." See vol. 45 on the "Miscellaneous Diseases of Small children," entry on "Vigorous Warmth."

（一）上八味，咬咀，以水四升，煮竹葉、　　小
　　　麥，取三升。去竹葉、　麥，下諸藥，煮取
　　　一升半，分三服。

（二）若小兒夏月忽壯熱燒人手，洞下黃溏，氣
　　　力惙然，脈極洪數，用此方加大黃二兩，
　　　再服，得下即瘥。

Preparation

(1) Pound the eight ingredients above. Decoct the *zhúyè* and *xiǎomài* in 4 *shēng* of water until reduced to 3 *shēng*. Remove the *zhúyè* and *xiǎomài*, add all the other medicinals, and decoct until reduced to 1.5 *shēng*. Divide into three doses.

(2) If a small child during the summer months suddenly [suffers from] vigorous heat hot enough to burn someone's hand, with yellow sloppy through-flux diarrhea, depleted energy, and an extremely surging and rapid pulse, use this formula with the addition of 2 *liǎng* of *dàhuáng*, divided into two doses. Once you have achieved a downward movement, recovery will ensue.

竹葉湯

主五六歲兒溫壯，腹中急滿，息不利，或有微腫。亦主極羸，不下飲食，堅癖，手足逆冷竹葉湯方。

竹葉	切，一升
小麥	半升
甘草	各二兩
黃芩	二銖
栝蔞根	
澤瀉	
茯苓	
知母	
白朮	
大黃	
桂心	
生薑	一兩半
人參	各一兩
麥門冬	
半夏	
當歸	十八銖

上十六味，咬咀，以水七升，煮小麥、竹葉，取四升，去滓，納藥，煎取一升六合，分四服。

V.14.b Zhúyè Tāng (Bamboo Leaf Decoction), Version Two

Indication

A formula indicated for vigorous warmth in children five to six *suì* old, with tension and fullness in the abdomen, inhibited breathing, and possibly mild swelling. It is also indicated for extreme emaciation, failure to get down food or drink, hardness and *pǐ* glomus, and counterflow cold in the hands and feet.

Ingredients

zhúyè	chopped, 1 *shēng*
xiǎomài	0.5 *shēng*
gāncǎo	
huángqín	
guālóugēn	
zéxiè	
fúlíng	2 *liǎng* each
zhīmǔ	
báizhú	
dàhuáng	
guìxīn	2 *zhū*
shēngjiāng	1.5 *liǎng*
rénshēn	
màiméndōng	1 *liǎng* each
bànxià	
dāngguī	18 *zhū*

Preparation

Pound the sixteen ingredients above. Cook the *xiǎomài* and *zhúyè* in 7 *shēng* of water until reduced to 4 *shēng*. Remove the dregs, add the various medicinals, and simmer until reduced to 1 *shēng* and 6 *gě*. Divide into four doses.

小兒連壯熱，實滯不去，寒熱往來，微驚悸方。

大黃	一兩
黃芩	各十八銖
栝蔞根	
甘草	
桂心	半兩
滑石	二兩
牡蠣	各半兩
人參	
龍骨	
凝水石	
白石脂	
硝石	

（一）上十二味，咬咀，以水四升，煮取一升半。

（二）服三合，一日一夜令盡，雖吐亦與之。

V.14.c Unnamed Formula for Vigorous Warmth

Indication
A formula for continuous vigorous heat in small children, with repletion and stagnation that cannot be eliminated, intermittent cold and heat, and mild fright palpitations.

Ingredients

dàhuáng	1 *liǎng*
huángqín	18 *zhū* each
guālóugēn	
gāncǎo	
guìxīn	0.5 *liǎng*
huáishí	2 *liǎng*
mǔlì	0.5 *liǎng* each
rénshēn	
lónggǔ	
níngshuǐshí	
báishízhī	
xiāoshí	

Editorial comment: Another edition adds 0.5 *liǎng* of *zǐshíyīng*.

Preparation
(1) Pound the twelve ingredients above and decoct in 4 *shēng* of water until reduced to 1.5 *shēng*.

(2) Take 3 *gě* per dose, using it all up in a single day and night. Even if the patient vomits, continue giving it.

《衍義》

（一）《千金》治五心煩熱，口乾脣燥，胸中熱悶，有竹葉湯。

（二）方用竹葉、小麥、知母、石膏、茯苓、麥冬、人參、甘草、栝蔞、半夏、生薑。

（三）其第一方南陽竹葉石膏中去石膏、半夏、粳米，加小麥、茯苓、黃芩、柴胡。

（四）蓋竹葉石膏湯本治傷寒解後，虛羸少氣，氣逆欲吐，故用石膏、粳米以清胃中餘熱，半夏以治氣逆欲吐。

（五）設無吐逆，可無藉於半夏也。

（六）此治小兒腹中伏熱，溫壯往來，故用小麥、茯苓以除伏熱煩擾，黃芩、柴胡以治溫壯來往。

Formulas for Vigorous Warmth Yǎn Yì (Expanded Meaning)

(1) There is a formula for Zhúyè Tāng [elsewhere] in the *Qiān Jīn Fāng* that treats vexing heat in the five hearts, dry mouth and lips, and heat and oppression in the chest.

(2) That formula uses *zhúyè, xiǎomài, zhīmǔ, shígāo, fúlíng, màiméndōng, rénshēn, gāncǎo, guālóugēn, bànxià*, and *shēngjiāng*.

(3) The first formula above is [created on the basis of] Zhāng Zhòngjǐng's Zhúyè Shígāo Tāng, but with *shígāo, bànxià*, and *jīngmǐ* removed and *xiǎomài, fúlíng, huángqín*, and *cháihú* added.

(4) Now Zhúyè Shígāo Tāng originally is a treatment for vacuity emaciation, shortage of qì, qì counterflow, and impending vomiting in cases of cold damage after it has been resolved. Therefore it uses *shígāo* and *jīngmǐ* to clear the residual heat in the stomach, and *bànxià* to treat the qì counterflow and impending vomiting.

(5) If there is no vomiting and counterflow, we do not need to make use of *bànxià*.

(6) The present formula [under discussion here] treats deep-lying heat inside the abdomen in small children, with intermittently occurring vigorous warmth. Therefore it uses *xiǎomài* and *fúlíng* to eliminate the vexation and harassment from the deep-lying heat, and *huángqín* and *cháihú* to treat the intermittently occurring vigorous warmth.

（七）設無溫壯，可無藉於柴胡也。

（八）其又方，但於前方除去柴胡一味，仍用竹葉石膏湯中知母、半夏，加入白朮、大黃、桂心、當歸、栝蔞根、澤瀉，生薑。

（九）其妙用全在桂心一味。

（十）知母、黃芩得之以破其結，大黃、白朮得之以振其威。

（十一）奇兵妙用，洵非庸俗可得而擬議者。

（十二）其三方，治小兒連壯熱實滯即又方之變法。

（十三）其用石脂、龍骨、牡蠣即又方白朮之意，用滑石即又方澤瀉之意，用凝水石即又方竹葉、知母之意，用硝石即又半夏、生薑之意。

（十四）不特能滌痰涎，兼可助桂心，為祛熱之嚮導也。

(7) If there is no vigorous warmth, we do not need to make use of *cháihú*.

(8) The second formula above has merely eliminated the single ingredient *cháihú* from the previous formula, but still uses the ingredients *zhīmǔ* and *bànxià* from Zhúyè Shígāo Tāng, with the addition of *báizhú, dàhuáng, guìxīn, dāngguī, guālóugēn, zéxiè,* and *shēngjiāng*.

(9) Its ingenious effect rests entirely on the single ingredient *guìxīn*.

(10) *Zhīmǔ* and *huángqín* are used to break up the binds, while *dàhuáng* and *báizhú* are used to arouse the power [of the medicinal preparation].

(11) This ingenious deployment of surprise troops is truly a scheme devised in a way that is unattainable by ordinary minds.

(12) The third formula here, which treats continuous vigorous heat in small children with repletion and stagnation, is in fact simply a variation on the second formula.

(13) Its use of *shízhī, lónggǔ,* and *mǔlì* has the same intention as that of *báizhú* in the second formula. Its use of *huáishí* has the same intention as that of *zéxiè* in that formula. Its use of *níngshuǐshí* has the same intention as that of *zhúyè* and *zhīmǔ* in that formula. And its use of *xiāoshí* has the same intention as that of *bànxià* and *shēngjiāng* there.

(14) Not only is it able to flush out phlegm-drool, but it is at the same time able to assist *guìxīn* and serves to lead the way in dispelling heat.

調中湯

治小兒春秋月晨夕中暴冷，冷氣折其四肢，熱不得泄，則壯熱，冷氣入胃，變下痢，或欲赤白滯起數去，小腹脹痛，極壯熱，氣脈洪大，或急數者，服之熱便歇，下亦瘥也，但壯熱不吐下者，亦主之方。

葛根	
黃芩	
茯苓	
桔梗	
芍藥	各六銖
白朮	
藁本	
大黃	
甘草	

（一）上九味，㕮咀，以水二升，煮取五合。

（二）服如後法：

V.15 Tiáo Zhōng Tāng (Center-Attuning Decoction)

Indication

A formula for small children, to treat fulminant cold at dawn and dusk during the spring and fall months, with cold qì folding over the extremities and heat that the patient is unable to discharge, resulting in vigorous heat, cold qì entering the stomach and transforming into diarrhea, possibly impending red or white [feces] that begin sluggishly but end with numerous bowel movements, Distension and pain in the lesser abdomen, extremely vigorous heat, and a qì flow in the vessels that is surging and large or urgent and rapid. When the patient takes this medicine, the heat will cease and the [pathological] bowel movements will also be cured. In cases of severe heat alone but without vomiting and [pathological] bowel movements, this formula is indicated as well.

Ingredients

gégēn	
huángqín	
fúlíng	
jiégěng	
sháoyào	6 *zhū* each
báizhú	
gǎoběn	
dàhuáng	
gāncǎo	

Preparation

(1) Pound the nine ingredients above and decoct in 2 *shēng* of water until reduced to 5 *gě*.

(2) Take this medicine according to the following method:

（三）兒生一日至七日，取一合分三服。生八日
　　至十五日，取一合半分三服。生十六日至
　　二十日，取二合分三服。生二十日至三十
　　日，取三合分三服。生三十日至四十日，
　　取五合分三服。恐吃五合未得，更斟酌
　　之。其百日至三百日兒，一如前篇龍膽湯
　　加之。

調中湯《衍義》

（一）葛根、藁本、甘草，解表藥也。

（二）黃芩、芍藥、甘草，清熱藥也。

（三）大黃、黃芩、甘草，攻裡藥也。

（四）苓、朮、桔梗、甘草，和中藥也。

（五）為小兒寒鬱熱邪，腹痛下痢之的方，功用
　　與人參敗毒相仿。

(3) For a child between one and seven days old, take 1 *gě*, divided into three doses. For a child between eight and fifteen days old, take 1.5 *gě*, divided into three doses. For [a child] between sixteen and twenty days old, take 2 *gě*, divided into three doses. For [a child] between twenty and thirty days old, take 3 *gě*, divided into three doses. For [a child] between thirty and forty days old, take 5 *gě*, divided into three doses. If you fear that consuming 5 *gě* has not achieved [the desired results], change [the dosage] at your discretion. For a child between a hundred and three hundred days old, increase [the dosage] as described in the section on Lóngdǎn Tāng above.

Tiáo Zhōng Tāng (Center-Attuning Decoction) *Yǎn Yì* (Expanded Meaning)

(1) *Gégēn, gǎoběn,* and *gāncǎo* are medicinals that resolve the exterior.

(2) *Huángqín, sháoyào,* and *gāncǎo* are medicinals that clear heat.

(3) *Dàhuáng, huángqín,* and *gāncǎo* are medicinals that attack the interior.

(4) *Fúlíng, báizhú, jiégěng,* and *gāncǎo* are medicinals that harmonize the center.

(5) This is a formula for small children, to treat cold oppressively constraining heat evil, causing abdominal pain and diarrhea. Its use of attack is similar to the action of *rénshēn* in vanquishing toxin.

鬱

Commentary V.15 ✤ **Sabine Wilms**

鬱 *Yù:* translated in Wiseman's Practical Dictionary of Chinese Medicine as "depression," this character is most familiar to contemporary practitioners of Chinese medicine in the compound 肝氣鬱 *gān qì yù,* for which the standard translation is "Liver Qi Stagnation." It is quite likely that what I consider a mis-translation of 鬱 as "stagnation" is based on it being confused with the character *yū* 瘀, which does mean "stasis" (as in the common compound 血瘀 "blood stasis"). Incidentally, that character is actually explained in the *Shuōwén Jiězì* as 積血 "accumulating blood." Returning to the character 鬱, however, which is pronounced in fourth tone and has absolutely no relationship to the character 瘀 (pronounced in first tone), it is a depiction of a pitcher surrounded by trees, on top of a roof, with sacrificial wine and radiance of light underneath. It thus conveys the idea of exuberant growth of vegetation to the point that it is covering up the light, as on the floor of a jungle or thicket. Gloominess and depression can be a connotation of this character, especially in certain modern compounds like 憂鬱 *yōuyù,* but our contemporary use of the term "depression," especially in medical contexts, is misleading and inaccurate. It literally refers to a pathological state where the qì is entangled, pent down or in, strangling and constraining itself like a root-bound plant in need of being freed from its container, unable to expand outwards freely, as it should in its healthy state. I have therefore chosen to translate it as "oppressive constraint."

生地黃湯

治小兒寒熱進退，啼呼腹痛方。

生地黃	各二兩
桂心	

（一）上二味，咬咀，以水三升，煮取一升。

（二）期歲以下服二合，以上三合。

V.16 Shēngdìhuáng Tāng (Raw Rehmannia Decoction)

Indication

A formula for small children, to treat advancing and retreating [aversion to] cold and heat [effusion] with crying and abdominal pain.

Ingredients

shēngdìhuáng	2 *liǎng* each
guìxīn	

Editorial comment: An alternative version of this formula contains seven ingredients, including 0.5 *liǎng* each of *sháoyào*, *hánshuǐshí, huángqín, dāngguī,* and *gāncǎo.*

Preparation

(1) Pound the two ingredients above and decoct in 3 *shēng* of water until reduced to 1 *shēng.*

(2) For children less than a full year old, give 2 *gě* per dose; for older children, give 3 *gě.*

生地黃湯《衍義》

（一）熱邪入犯營血，則寒熱進退。

（二）故用生地黃專治血熱，則兼桂心以行地黃
　　　之滯。

（三）寒熱兼濟之妙，無逾於此。

（四）又方合黃芩湯，則專主太陽少陽合病。

（五）更加寒水石以治心胃之火，當歸以散肝脾
　　　之熱也。

Shēngdìhuáng Tāng (Raw Rehmannia Decoction)
Yǎn Yì (Expanded Meaning)

(1) When heat evil has invaded the level of *yíng* provisioning and blood, the result is increasing and abating cold
and heat

(2) Therefore [the present formula] uses *shēngdìhuáng* to
specifically treat blood heat. This is then combined with
guìxīn to move the stagnation [potentially induced by]
dìhuáng.

(3) Nothing surpasses [this formula's] ingenuity in rescu-
ing [the patient] from cold and heat simultaneously.

(4) The second formula[16] combines [the first formula] with
Huángqín Tāng. Consequently, it is indicated specifically for combined Tàiyáng and Shàoyáng conditions.

(5) It further adds *hánshuǐshí* to treat the fire in the heart
and stomach, and *dāngguī* to disperse the heat in the
liver and spleen.

---

16   This is a reference to the formula variation with the five added ingredients that is mentioned in the editorial comment.

（一）治小兒傷寒發黃方：搗土瓜根汁三合，服之。

（二）又方：搗韭根汁，澄清，以滴兒鼻中，如大豆許，即出黃水瘥。

（三）又方：搗青麥汁，服之。

又方：

小豆	三七枚
瓜蒂	十四枚
糯米	四十粒

上三味，為末，吹鼻中。

V.17 Formulas for Cold Damage with Jaundice

(1) A formula for cold damage with jaundice in small children: Pound *tǔguāgēn* until you have 3 *gě* of juice. Make [the patient] ingest this.

(2) Another formula: Pound *jiǔgēn* to get the juice, [let the impurities] settle until [the juice] is clear, and drip it into the child's nose, in amounts roughly equal to a soybean. [When the child] now produces a discharge of a yellow liquid, this means recovery.

(3) Another formula: Pound green wheat[17] to get the juice. Make [the patient] ingest this.

Another formula:
Ingredients

xiǎodòu	3x7 pieces*
guādì	14 pieces
nuòmǐ	40 grains

*Translator's note: In other words, 21.

Preparation
Pulverize the three ingredients above and blow it up the [patient's] nose.

---

17   The exact identity of 青麥 *qīng mài* is uncertain, which is why I have translated it literally. It is mentioned in the *Shèng Jì Zǒng Lù* as a treatment for jaundice in small children. My best guess is that it might be the juice produced by squeezing sprouted wheat that has already turned green.

《衍義》

（一）土瓜根專主濕熱發黃。

（二）韭汁專散瘀熱。

（三）青麥汁專散肝熱。

（四）瓜蒂散加糯米吹鼻，取下黃水，專散在土濕熱也。

（五）但不可以筒極力過吹入腦，令人喘息立死。

Yǎn Yì (Expanded Meaning)

(1) *Tǔguāgēn* is indicated specifically for jaundice related damp heat.

(2) *Jiǔgēn* juice specifically disperses stasis heat.

(3) Green wheat juice specifically disperses liver heat.

(4) *Guādì* powder with the addition of *nuòmǐ*, blown up the nose, brings down yellow liquid and specifically disperses damp heat that is located in [spleen-]earth.

(5) Nevertheless, you must not use a tube and excessive force to blow it beyond [the nose] into the brain. This will cause the person to gasp for air and die instantly.

二物通汗散

治少小有熱不汗方。

雷丸	四兩
粉	半斤

上搗和，下篩，以粉兒身。

二物茯苓粉散

治少小頭汗方。

茯苓	各四兩
牡蠣	

上治下篩，以粉八兩，合搗為散，有熱輒以粉，汗即自止。

V.18 Formulas for Night Sweating

V.18.a Èr Wù Tōng Hàn Sǎn (Two-Ingredients Sweat-Freeing Powder)

Indication

A formula for children, to treat presence of heat without sweating.

Ingredients

léiwán	4 *liǎng*
rice powder	0.5 *jīn*

Preparation

Pound and mix the ingredients above and sift through a sieve. Sprinkle the powder on the child's body.

V.18.b Èr Wù Fúlíng Fěn Sǎn (Two-Ingredients Poria Powder)

Indication

A formula for children, to treat sweating from the head.

Ingredients

fúlíng	4 *liǎng* each
mǔlì	

Preparation

Finely pestle and sift the above ingredients. Combine with 8 *liǎng* of rice flour and pound into a powder. When there is heat, immediately sprinkle the powder on [the patient], and the sweating will stop spontaneously.

三物黄連粉

治少小盗汗方。

黄連	
牡蠣	各十八銖
貝母	

上以粉一升，合搗，下篩，以粉身良。

《衍義》

（一）雷丸殺三蟲，逐毒氣，去胃中熱，故能通汗。

（二）茯苓守五臟之氣。

（三）牡蠣斂下焦之熱。

（四）黄連、貝母寒潤，得牡蠣之咸寒。

（五）雜粉以粉兒身，專主小兒虛熱，津液不固之盗汗。

V.18.c Sān Wù Huánglián Fěn (Three-Ingredients Coptis Powder)

Indication

A formula to treat night sweating in children.

Ingredients

huánglián	
mǔlì	18 *zhū* each
bèimǔ	

Preparation

Combine the above ingredients with 1 *shēng* of rice flour and pound and sift them. Sprinkling this on the body is excellent.

Yǎn Yì (Expanded Meaning) (Commentary on Formulas for Night Sweating)

(1) *Léiwán* kills the three types of worms,[18] expels toxic qì, and gets rid of heat inside the stomach. Therefore it is able to open up the flow of sweat.

(2) *Fúlíng* safeguards the qì of the five *zàng* organs.

3) *Mǔlì* restrains heat in the Lower Burner.

(4) *Huánglián* and *bèimǔ* are cold and moistening and [are a good match] for the salty cold of *mǔlì*.

(5) Sprinkling these various powders on the child's body is indicated specifically for vacuity heat in small children [manifesting in] night sweating related to insecurity of the fluids.

---

18 三蟲 *sān chóng*: The three kinds of intestinal parasites common in small children, namely roundworms, intestinal flukes, and pinworms

犀角飲子

此由心臟熱之所感，宜服犀角飲子方。

犀角	十八銖
茯神	一兩
麥門冬	一兩半
甘草	半兩
白朮	六銖

上五味，咬咀，以水九合，煎取四合，分服。加龍齒一兩佳。

犀角飲子《衍義》

（一）犀角散熱之首藥。

（二）得門冬、茯神引入心包，白朮、甘草斂津液。

（三）倘服之不應加龍齒以收肝氣之散。

V.19 Xījiǎo Yǐnzǐ (Rhinoceros Horn Drink)

Indication

When this [night sweating] is caused by a contraction of heat in the heart *zàng* organ, it is suitable to give this formula.

Ingredients

xījiǎo	18 *zhū*
fúshén	1 *liǎng*
màiméndōng	1.5 *liǎng*
gāncǎo	0.5 *liǎng*
báizhú	6 *zhū*

Preparation

Pound the five ingredients above and decoct in 9 *gě* of water until reduced to 4 *gě*. Divide into doses. Adding 1 *liǎng* of *lóng-chǐ* is excellent.

Xījiǎo Yǐnzǐ (Rhinoceros Horn Drink)
***Yǎn Yì* (Expanded Meaning)**

(1) *Xījiǎo* is the foremost medicinal for dispersing heat.

(2) It is here matched with *màiméndōng* and *fúshén*, which draw it into the pericardium, and with *báizhú* and *gāncǎo*, which hold in the fluids.

(3) If you do not get a response after taking it, add *lóngchǐ* to gather in the dispersal of liver qì.

恆山湯

治小兒溫瘧方。

恆山	一兩，切
小麥	三合
淡竹葉	切，一升

（一）上三味，以水一升半，煮取五合。

（二）一日至七日兒，一合為三服。八日至十五日兒，一合半為三服。十六日至二十日兒，二合為三服。四十日至六十日兒，六合為三服。六十日至百日兒，一服二合半。百日至二百日兒，一服三合。

恆山湯《衍義》

（一）恒山專滌內蘊之痰，為截瘧之峻味。

（二）小麥、竹葉專清胃中煩熱也。

V.20 Héngshān Tāng (Dichroa Decoction)

Indication
A formula for small children to treat warm malaria.

Ingredients

héngshān	1 *liǎng*, chopped
xiǎomài	3 *gě*
dànzhúyè	chopped, 1 *shēng*

Preparation
(1) Decoct the three ingredients above in 1.5 *shēng* of water until reduced to 5 *gě*.

(2) In children one to seven days old, give 1 *gě* in three doses. In children eight to fifteen days old, give 1.5 *gě* in three doses. In children sixteen to twenty days old, give 2 *gě* in three doses. In children forty to sixty days old, give 6 *gě* in three doses. In children sixty to a hundred days old, give 2.5 *gě* per dose. In children one to two hundred days old, give 3 *gě* per dose.

Héngshān Tāng (Dichroa Decoction)
***Yǎn Yì* (Expanded Meaning)**

(1) *Héngshān* specifically flushes out internally smoldering phlegm. It is a fierce ingredient for interrupting malaria.

(2) *Xiǎomài* and *zhúyè* specifically clear the vexing heat inside the stomach.

（一）又方：鹿角末，臨發時先服一錢匕。

（二）又方：燒鱉甲灰，以酒服一錢匕，至發時服三匕，並以火灸身。

（三）又方：燒雞膍胵中黃皮，末，和乳與服，男雄女雌。

《衍義》

（一）鹿角專補督脈，督脈固，則外邪不能容矣。

（二）鱉甲專闢肝邪，雞胵胵專滌胃滯，肝胃淨，寒熱自除。

小兒溫瘧，灸兩乳下一指三壯。

V.21 Formulas for Malaria

(1) Another formula: Pulverize *lùjiǎo* and give 1 *qián*-spoon right before it is about to erupt.

(2) Another formula: Char *biējiǎ* into ashes and give 1 *qián*-spoon in liquor. Right at the onset of an attack, give three spoons. At the same time, "roast" the body by the fire.

(3) Another formula: Char the lining of a chicken's gizzard[19] and pulverize it. Have the child take it mixed into [breast] milk. For boys, use a rooster's; for girls, a hen's.

---

19   This ingredient is more commonly referred to as *jīnèijīn*.

Yǎn Yì (Expanded Meaning) (Commentary on Malaria Formulas)

(1) *Lùjiǎo* specifically supplements the Dūmài (Governing Vessel). When the Dūmài is secured, external evils cannot be contained therein!

(2) *Biējiǎ* specifically repels evils from the liver, while chicken's gizzard lining specifically flushes out stagnation from the stomach. When the liver and stomach are cleansed, cold and heat will be eliminated spontaneously.

V.22 Moxibustion

For warm malaria in small children, burn three cones of moxa one finger-width below both nipples.

CHAPTER SIX: COUGH

咳嗽第六

(14 formulas)

竹瀝湯

（一）小兒出胎二百許日，頭身患小小瘡，治護
小瘥，複發，五月中忽小小咳嗽，微溫和
治之。

（二）因變癇，一日二十過發，四肢縮動，背脊(
身天)　　肭，眼反，須臾氣絕，良久複
蘇，已與常治癇湯，得快吐下，經日不
間。

（三）爾後單與竹瀝汁。　稍進，一日一夕中合進
一升許，發時小疏。

（四）明日與此竹瀝湯，得吐下，發便大折，其
間猶稍稍與竹瀝汁。

Commentary VI.1.a ᴕ **Sabine Wilms**

The use of the character 發 *fā* is quite evocative here. Usually
translated as "to emit, express, expose" or "to rise" (as in the fer-
mentation process), in the medical context it carries the specific
meaning of something coming to the surface and erupting from
there. I therefore translate it as "eruption" or "outbreak." This
meaning is reflected in such common compounds as 發熱 *fā rè* (lit.
"eruption of heat," i.e. fever), 發病 *fā bìng* (the onset of a disease),
or 發汗 *fā hàn* (to induce sweating). In the present context, the fetal
toxin (胎毒 *tāi dú*) is coming to the surface, figuratively and literally, in several stages of progressing severity, erupting first as a
classic measles-type skin rash, then as coughing with a mild temperature, and lastly as severe seizures with loss of consciousness.
Due to the underlying root cause of fetal toxin, it is not enough
in treatment to address the outward symptoms of the patient. In
addition, it is essential to rid the body of the toxin by aggressively
moving it out of the body, both upward through vomiting and
downward through urination and defecation.

VI.1 Formulas with *Máhuáng* and *Dàhuáng*

VI.1.a Zhúlì Tāng (Bamboo Sap Decoction)

Indication

(1) [This formula is indicated for] small children who suffered from tiny sores on their head and body within the first two hundred days or so after birth. After recovering slightly because they received [medical] treatment and care, the disease erupted again. In the fifth month, [such patients] suddenly suffered from minor coughing with mild warmth and were treated for this.

(2) Consequently, the condition transformed into seizures, with twenty or more episodes in a single day [that manifested with] contractions and stirring of the four limbs, bending over and straightening of the spine and back, upcast eyes, fainting in an instant, and regaining consciousness after a good long while. Afterwards, patients received frequent treatment with decoctions for seizures, which quickly induced vomiting and downward expulsion. [This situation has persisted] for days without interruption.

(3) In a situation like this, afterwards administer only bamboo sap (*zhúlìzhī*). Give it to them a little bit at a time, continuously throughout an entire day and night, to a total of roughly 1 *shēng*. The outbreaks [of the seizures] will become a little less frequent.

(4) On the next day, administer the present formula for Zhúlì Tāng. Once you have induced vomiting and downward expulsion, an eruption [of the disease] will then be followed by a great break. In between [the outbreaks of seizures], continue administering small amounts of bamboo sap.

竹瀝	五合
黃芩	三十銖
木防己	各六銖
羚羊角	
大黃	二兩
茵芋	三銖
麻黃	各半兩
白薇	
桑寄生	
草薢	
甘草	
白朮	六銖

（一）上十二味，咬咀，以水二升半，煮取藥減
半，納竹瀝，煎取一升。

（二）分服二合，相去一食久，進一服。

Ingredients

zhúlì	5 *gě*
huángqín	30 *zhū*
mùfángjǐ	6 *zhū* each
língyángjiǎo	
dàhuáng	2 *liǎng*
yīnyù	3 *zhū*
máhuáng	0.5 *liǎng* each
báiwēi	
sāngjìshēng	
bìxiè	
gāncǎo	
báizhú	6 *zhū*

Editorial comments: Another version does not contain *bìxiè*.
Another version of this formula calls for *báixiān*.

Preparation

(1) Of the twelve ingredients above, pound [the dried herbs] and decoct in 2.5 *shēng* of water until the medicine is reduced to half. Add the *zhúlì* and decoct until reduced to 1 *shēng*.

(2) Divide it into doses of 2 *gě* and space them by the length of time it takes to eat a meal, then make the patient take another dose.

竹瀝湯《衍義》

（一）咳嗽有六淫七情，經絡臟腑，種種不侔。

（二）此專因胎毒發瘡後變發癇。

（三）與竹瀝治痰滌熱，雖得小疏，然非吐下不能大朽其勢。

（四）故用麻黃、白薇開發肺氣於上，即用大黃、黃芩、竹瀝疏利大腸於下。

（五）羚羊、防己、萆薢、寄生、茵芋專為熱毒發癇而設。

（六）白朮、甘草和中實脾，師旅之糧餉也。

Commentary VI.1.a ᴥ Julian Scott

I think this may well refer to measles, which in the developed world is now less dangerous than flu. In Third World countries, however, measles-related pneumonia is still the biggest single cause of infant mortality. Many years ago I used to treat measles regularly, and delirium and mild convulsions were still a possibility. In that case, the "tiny sores" could be interpreted as the spots that appear in measles.

At the time this was written, measles was considered entirely due to fetal poisons. There is apparently no reference to any wind component until there was contact with the West.

It is also true that if the measles rash does not come out properly, it can return again and again.

Zhúlì Tāng (Bamboo Sap Decoction) *Yǎn Yì* (Expanded Meaning)

(1) Cough has all sorts of different [etiologies], including the six excesses and seven emotions,[1] the channels and network vessels, and the viscera and bowels.

(2) The present formula specifically [addresses cases of cough] caused by fetal toxin that erupted as sores and afterwards transformed to erupt as seizures.

(3) Administering bamboo sap treats phlegm and flushes out heat. While [this treatment] does achieve a minor reduction in the frequency [of outbreaks], without inducing vomiting and downward expulsion you will not be able to substantially break its might.

(4) For this reason, the formula uses *máhuáng* and *báiwēi* to open up and effuse lung qì upward, and uses *dàhuáng*, *huángqín*, and *zhúlì* to course and disinhibit the large intestine downward.

(5) *Língyáng*, *fángjǐ*, *bìxiè*, *jìshēng*, and *yīnyù* are intended here specifically to address the heat toxin that is erupting as seizures.

(6) *Báizhú* and *gāncǎo* harmonize the center and make the spleen replete, serving as army provisions for the entirety of troops.

---

1 Both of these phrases are technical terms with specific meanings in medical literature: In the context of pathogenesis in particular, the six excesses (六淫 *liù yín*) refers to the six environmental causes of diease, -- wind, cold, fire, summerheat, dampness, and dryness,-- while the seven emotions (七情 *qī qíng*) refers to the internal causes of disease -- joy, anger, anxiety, overthinking, sorrow, fear, and fright.

紫菀湯

治小兒中冷及傷寒暴嗽，或上氣，咽喉鳴，氣
逆，或鼻塞，清水出者方。

紫菀	各半兩
杏仁	
麻黃	各六銖
桂心	
橘皮	
青木香	
黃芩	各半兩
當歸	
甘草	
大黃	一兩

（一）上十味，㕮咀，以水三升，煮取九合，去
　　滓。

（二）六十日至百日兒，一服二合半。一百日至
　　二百日兒，一服三合。

VI.1.b Zǐwǎn Tāng (Aster Decoction)

Indication

A formula for small children, to treat fulminant coughing from cold strike and cold damage, possibly with qì ascent, throat rale, and qì counterflow, or with nasal congestion and clear discharge.

Ingredients

zǐwǎn	0.5 *liǎng* each
xìngrén	
máhuáng	6 *zhū* each
guìxīn	
júpí	
qīngmùxiāng	
huángqín	0.5 *liǎng* each
dāngguī	
gāncǎo	
dàhuáng	1 *liǎng*

Preparation

(1) Pound the ten ingredients above and decoct in 3 *shēng* of water until reduced to 9 *gě*. Remove the dregs.

(2) For children between sixty and a hundred days old, give 2.5 *gě* per dose. For children between one and two hundred days old, give 3 *gě* per dose.

紫菀湯 《衍義》

（一）前方重在瘡毒發癇，故用羚羊、防己、茵
　　　芋等味。

（二）此方專主寒嗽，故取《古今錄驗》橘皮湯
　　　全方，但加大黃、青木香二味，以滌內積
　　　之乳癖。

（三）不可拘於大人治例也。

Commentary VI.1.b ◆ Sabine Wilms

As Dr. Julian Scott notes, "when babies and toddlers present with a cough, it is essential that we always look out for the possibility of food accumulations." Given the large number of formulas to treat "Aggregations, Binds, Distension, and Fullness" (see the following Chapter Seven, pp. 144-227) and the harsh nature of many of the formulas and ingredients used therein, the danger of food being retained instead of being properly digested and eliminated must have been a very important worry of medieval physicians in the treatment of small children. It presents an interesting contrast with Sūn Sīmiǎo's repeated warnings against overly invasive treatments, given the fragile health of newborns and small children (see *Venerating the Root, Part One*, chapter 1).

Zǐwǎn Tāng (Aster Decoction) *Yǎn Yì* (Expanded Meaning)

(1) The previous formula placed the emphasis on sores, [fetal] toxin, and the eruption of seizures. Hence it used ingredients like *língyáng*, *fángjǐ*, and *yīnyù*.

(2) The present formula is indicated specifically for cold[-related] cough and hence takes the entire formula for Júpí Tāng from the *Gǔjīn Lù Yàn*. It only adds the two ingredients *dàhuáng* and *qīngmùxiāng*, to sweep away the milk aggregations that have accumulated inside.[2]

(3) This is a treatment precedent that we must not restrict to adults alone.

---

2   According to Julian Scott, when babies and toddlers get a cough, one always has to look out for the possibility of food accumulation.

Commentary VI.1.b ✴ Sabine Wilms (continued)

A similar dichotomy between general words of caution, followed by what strikes us modern readers as dangerously strong formulas in the clinical part of the text can be found in the volumes on gynecology. Most likely, these opposing sentiments reflect either two different sources that Sun Simiao relied on to compose this text, or the fact that he composed the essays himself but followed up with all the formulas that he could gather from various textual or oral sources. In this context, it is also important to remember that the title of this entire book includes the reference to "prepare for emergence" (備急 *bèi jí*) and that the text was created at a time without ambulances, antibiotics, major surgical interventions, and Emergency facilities.

五味子湯

治小兒風冷入肺，上氣氣逆，面青，喘迫咳嗽，晝夜不息，食則吐不下方。

五味子	各半兩
當歸	
麻黃	各兩銖
乾薑	
桂心	
人參	
紫菀	
甘草	
細辛	各三銖
款冬花	
大黃	一兩半

（一）上十一味，㕮咀，以水二升半，煮取九合，去滓。

（二）兒六十日至百日，一服二合半。一百日至二百日，一服三合。

（三）其大黃別浸一宿下。

VI.1.c Wǔwèizǐ Tāng (Schisandra Decoction)

Indication

A formula for small children, to treat wind and coolness entering the lung, with ascent of qì and qì counterflow, a green-blue face, panting in distress and coughing that does not stop day or night, and vomiting and inability to move food down upon eating.

Ingredients

wǔwèizǐ	0.5 *liǎng* each
dāngguī	
máhuáng	2 *zhū* each
gānjiāng	
guìxīn	
rénshēn	
zǐwǎn	
gāncǎo	
xìxīn	3 *zhū* each
kuǎndōnghuā	
dàhuáng	3 *zhū* each

Editorial comment: An alternative [version of this] formula does not contain *kuǎndōnghuā* or *dàhuáng* but contains three pieces of *dàzǎo*.

Preparation

(1) Pound the eleven ingredients above and decoct in 2.5 *shēng* of water until reduced to 9 *gě*. Remove the dregs.

(2) For children between sixty and a hundred days old, give 2.5 *gě* per dose. For children between a hundred and two hundred days old, a dose is 3 *gě*.

(3) Do not soak the *dàhuáng* for less than one full night.

五味子湯《衍義》

（一）小兒風冷入肺咳嗽，用麻、桂、姜、辛、
　　　款冬、甘、苑當矣。

（二）以其有面青喘迫，吐逆不下，知肺胃之氣
　　　大虛。

（三）非藉人參，不能安其胃氣，非藉白朮，不
　　　能止其吐逆，非藉五味，不能斂其喘迫。

（四）蓋小兒面青逆冷，必非伏熱假象，但其咳
　　　嗽晝夜不息，必有乳癖留滯於中。

（五）若係虛嗽，火動則劇，火靜則止，定屬虛
　　　中挾痰之象無疑。

（六）非藉大黃不能滌其乳癖，非藉當歸不能和
　　　其血氣。

（七）上三方，總藉麻黃、大黃，內外上下兼並
　　　之力也。

Wǔwèizǐ Tāng (Schisandra Decoction) *Yǎn Yì* (Expanded Meaning)

(1) For small children with wind and coolness enter-ing the lung and causing cough, the use of *máhuáng*, *guìxīn*, *gānjiāng*, *xìxīn*, *kuǎndōnghuā*, *gāncǎo*, and *zǐwǎn* is compelling.

(2) Based on the fact that [the patient] is presenting with a green-blue face, panting in distress, and vomiting with counterflow and inability to move [food] downward, we know that the qì of the lung and stomach is greatly vacuous.

(3) Without relying on *rénshēn*, we would be unable to set the patient's stomach qì at ease. Without relying on *báizhú*, we would be unable to stop the patient's vomit-ing and counterflow. And without relying on *wǔwèizǐ*, we would be unable to control the patient's distressed panting.

(4) Now, in small children a green-blue face with coun-terflow coolness can never be a false manifestation of deep-lying heat. Instead, the coughing that continues day and night without stopping must mean the pres-ence of milk aggregations stagnating in the center.

(5) If this condition were related to vacuity cough, it would be aggravated when the fire is active but stop when the fire calms down. Hence it is certain that [the present condition] is associated with manifestations of vacuity that is complicated by phlegm. There is no doubt.

Commentary VI.1.c ◀ Sabine Wilms

The specific warning against decocting the *dàhuáng* for an insufficient amount of time is based on the fact that its downwardly expelling action would otherwise be too drastic for a small child and therefore has to be toned down by decocting it overnight. As described in the *Běncǎo Jīng*, "*Dàhuáng* pushes out the old and makes the new arrive" (大黃推陳致新). The applicability of this medicinal effect in the present context needs no further explanation. Similarly, the risk of employing such a strongly acting substance in the context of pediatric treatments should be obvious to any experienced practitioner. The vulnerability of the neonatal state is a theme that Sūn Sīmiǎo returns to again and again, and most likely the primary reason why he chose to place the section on pediatrics in the first part of his book, right after the section on gynecology and ahead of the general section.

(6) Without relying on *dàhuáng*, we would be unable to flush out the milk aggregations, and without relying on *dānggui*, we would be unable to harmonize the patient's blood and qì.

(7) The three formulas above all rely on *máhuáng* and *dàhuáng*, to combine their force internally and externally and above and below at the same time.

治小兒、大人咳逆短氣，胸中吸吸，呵出涕唾，嗽出臭膿方。

（一）燒淡竹瀝，煮二十沸。小兒一服一合，日
　　　五服。

（二）大人一升，亦日五服。

（三）不妨食息乳哺。

《衍義》

此即前第一方所言單與竹瀝汁之法也。

VI.2 Formulas for Counterflow Cough

VI.2.a
Indication

A formula for small children and adults, to treat counterflow cough with shortness of breath, heavy inhaling in the chest, exhaling with nasal and oral discharge, and coughing with foul-smelling pus.

Ingredients and Preparation

(1) Roast *dànzhú* [to get] the sap and decoct this, bringing it to a boil 20 times. For small children, give 1 *gě* per dose, 5 doses a day.

(2) For adults, give 1 *shēng* [per dose], and also give 5 doses per day.

(3) Do not impede feeding or stop nursing.

Yǎn Yì (Expanded Meaning)

This [treatment] is the method referenced in the very first formula above, which tells us to administer the single ingredient *zhúlì* juice as part of a multi-step treatment program.[3]

---

3   See above, section VI.1a, line 3.

治小兒寒熱咳逆，膈中有癖，乳若吐，不欲食
方。

乾地黃	四兩
麥門冬	各半斤
五味子	
蜜	
大黃	各一兩
硝石	

（一）上六味，㕮咀，以水三升，煮取一升，去
滓，納硝石、蜜，煮令沸。

（二）服二合，日三。

（三）胸中當有宿乳汁一升許也。

（四）大者服五合。

VI.2.b

A formula for small children, to treat cold and heat[4] and counterflow cough, with the presence of aggregations in the diaphragm, an appearance like vomiting when breastfeeding, and lack of appetite.[5]

Ingredients

gāndìhuáng	4 *liǎng*
màiméndōng	0.5 *jīn* each
wǔwèizǐ	
fēngmì	
dàhuáng	1 *liǎng* each
xiāoshí	

Preparation

(1) Of the six ingredients above, pound [the herbs] and decoct in 3 *shēng* of water until reduced to 1 *shēng*. Remove the dregs, add the *xiāoshí* and honey, and decoct it, bringing it to a boil.

(2) Give 2 *gě* per dose, 3 doses a day.

(3) In the center of the chest, there should be about 1 *shēng* of abiding breast milk [that the formula helps to expel].[6]

(4) For adult [patients], a dose is 5 *gě*.

---

4   Most commonly, 寒熱 means "cold and heat" in the sense of alternating aversion to cold and heat effusion. Given the location in the sentence, here, and the nature of the formula, however, it is quite possible that this phrase could mean "cold or heat" here, in other words that the formula treats counterflow cough that is occurring in conditions that are either predominantly cold or predominantly hot.

5   Translator's note: The *Yǎn Yì* edition of this text slightly changes the order of characters to 膈中有乳癖，若吐。。。 This would be translated as "...with the presence of milk aggregations, and an appearance like vomiting and lack of appetite."

6   The various editions differ quite substantially here. Some have 汗 *hàn* ("sweat") instead of 許 *xǔ* ("about"), and some have 出 *chū* ("expel") instead of 也 *yě* (sentence end particle). The meaning of this sentence remains the same, though, namely that there is an amount of about 1 *shēng* of abiding breast milk that has aggregated in the diaphragm and that needs to get expelled through the action of this formula, in order to treat this condition.

《衍義》

（一）地黃、麥冬、蜂蜜、五味治久咳肺燥。

（二）因膈中有乳癖，故用硝、黃，不用芒硝，
　　　而用硝石專磨乳癖之用也。

治小兒咳逆，喘息如水雞聲方。

射乾	一兩
半夏	五枚
桂心	五寸
麻黃	各一兩
紫菀	
甘草	
生薑	
大棗	二十枚

上八味，㕮咀，以水七升，煮取一升五合，去
滓，納蜜五合，煎一沸，分溫服二合，日三。

Yăn Yì (Expanded Meaning)

(1) *Dìhuáng, màiméndōng, fēngmì,* and *wǔwèizǐ* treat chronic cough with dryness in the lung.

(2) Because of the presence of milk aggregations in the diaphragm, the formula uses *xiāoshí* and *dàhuáng.* The reason why it does not use *mángxiāo* but uses *xiāoshí* instead is its specific effect of "grinding down" the milk aggregations.

VI.3 Formulas for Cough with Panting

VI.3.a Shègān Tāng (Belamcanda Decoction)

Indication

A formula for small children, to treat counterflow cough with gasping for breath and a frog-like rale in the throat.

Ingredients

shègān	1 *liǎng*
bànxià	5 pieces
guìxīn	5 *cùn*
máhuáng	1 *liǎng* each
zǐwǎn	
gāncǎo	
shēngjiāng	
dàzǎo	20 pieces

Preparation

Pound the eight ingredients above and decoct in 7 *shēng* of water until reduced to 1 *shēng* and 5 *gě.* Remove the dregs. Add 5 *gě* of honey and reheat, bringing it to a boil one more time. Divide and take warm in doses of 2 *gě,* 3 times a day.

射乾湯《衍義》

（一）此於《金匱》射乾麻黃湯中，除去細辛、
款冬、五味，易入桂心、甘草、蜂蜜。

（二）雖主治與《金匱》無異，而桂心和營，較
細辛搜肺之力稍緩，甘草和胃，較五味收
津之味稍平，蜂蜜潤燥，較款冬散結之性
稍和。

（三）非若前五味子湯之有面青喘迫，不得不藉
參、朮、五味之收斂津氣也。

Shègān Tāng (Belamcanda Decoction) Yǎn Yì (Expanded Meaning)

(1) This formula [is a modification of] Shègān Máhuáng Tāng from the *Jīn Guì Yào Lüè*, eliminating *xìxīn*, *kuǎndōnghuā*, and *wǔwèizǐ* and instead adding *guìxīn*, *gāncǎo*, and *fēngmì*.

(2) From [the indications of that formula in] the *Jīn Guì Yào Lüè*, [the effect of] *guìxīn* to harmonize the *yíng* provisioning level is a bit more moderate than the strength of *xìxīn* to rout [pathogenic factors] in the lung; the effect of *gāncǎo* to harmonize the stomach is a bit more balanced than the flavor of *wǔwèizǐ* to astringe liquids; and the action of *fēngmì* to moisten dryness is a bit more harmonious than the inherent nature of *kuǎndōnghuā* to disperse binds.

(3) [The condition for which] the present [formula is indicated] is not like the green-blue face and panting in distress [described above as the indication for] Wǔwèizǐ Tāng. [In that case,] you have no choice but must rely on [the effect of] *rénshēn*, *báizhú*, and *wǔwèizǐ* to gather in and astringe the liquids and qì.

又方

半夏	四兩
紫菀	二兩
款冬花	二合
蜜	一合
桂心	各二兩
生薑	
細辛	
阿膠	
甘草	

（一）上九味，㕮咀，以水七升，煮半夏，取六
升，去滓，納諸藥，煮取二升五合。

（二）五歲兒服一升，二歲兒服六合，量兒大小
多少加減之。

《衍義》

前方專搜風寒逆氣，此方專搜痰飲瘀結，雖所見
之證與前無異，而受病之源不侔也。

VI.3.b Another Formula

Ingredients

bànxià	4 *liǎng*
zǐwǎn	2 *liǎng*
kuǎndōnghuā	2 *gě*
mì	1 *gě*
guìxīn	
shēngjiāng	
xìxīn	2 *liǎng* each
ējiāo	
gāncǎo	

Preparation

(1) Pound the nine ingredients above. Decoct the *bànxià* in 7 *shēng*[7] until reduced to 6 *shēng* and remove the dregs. Add all the other medicinals and decoct until reduced to 2 *shēng* and 5 *gě*.

(2) For a child of five *suì*, give 1 *shēng* per dose. For a child of two *suì*, give 6 *gě* per dose. Increase or reduce the amount in accordance with the child's age.

---

7 A number of editions have 1 *shēng* here instead, obviously a textual error that is sometimes corrected, on the basis of yet other editions, as 1 *dǒu*.

Yǎn Yì (Expanded Meaning)

The previous formula specifically tracks down wind, cold, and counterflow qì. This present formula specifically tracks down phlegm rheum stasis binds. Even though the visible signs are no different from the previous formula, the source from which the disease was contracted is not the same.

杏仁丸

主大人、小兒咳逆上氣方。

杏仁	三升熟搗如膏
蜜	一升為三份

（一）以一份納杏仁搗，令強，更納一份搗之如膏，又納一份搗熟止。

（二）先食已含咽之，多少自在，日三。

（三）每服不得過半方寸匕，則利。

VI.3.c Xìngrén Wán (Apricot Pit Pill)

Indication

A formula for adults and small children alike, indicated for counterflow cough with ascent of qì.

Ingredients

xìngrén	3 *shēng*, thoroughly crushed into a paste-like consistency.
fēngmì	1 *shēng* divided into thirds.

Preparation

(1) Take one part [of the honey], add it to the apricot pits, and beat until stiff. Add another part and beat until it has a paste-like consistency. Then add the last part and beat until it is thoroughly [combined]. Then stop.

(2) Before meals, [have the patient] hold it in the mouth or throat and swallow it, in whatever amount is comfortable, three times a day.

(3) Each dose may not exceed half a square-*cùn* spoon full, or it will induce diarrhea.[8]

---

8   Some editions here have 痢 *lì* ("dysentery") instead of 利 *lì* ("diarrhea" or more generally "disinhibition"). In any case, the meaning is obviously that excessive amounts of *xìngrén* will act too harshly in inducing a bowel movement and should therefore be taken with caution.

杏仁丸《衍義》

（一）杏仁為辛散肺氣之峻藥。

（二）生用則治傷寒喘逆，熬黑則治結胸痰垢，其耗氣之性可知。

（三）此與蜜三份和搗，籍其甘溫潤澤，以降肺逆，可為曲盡制度之妙。

（四）然服不過半方寸匕則痢，使肺氣從大腸降泄。

（五）無復咳逆上氣之患矣。

Xìngrén Wán (Apricot Pit Pill) *Yǎn Yì* (Expanded Meaning)

(1) *Xìngrén* is a harshly-acting medicinal that disperses lung qì with acridity.

(2) Used raw, it treats cold damage with panting and counterflow. Simmered until black, it treats phlegm and filth binding in the chest. Its characteristic of wearing on [the patient's] qì is well-known.

(3) Combining it with honey and beating it in in three parts relies on the sweet warm moistening [properties of the honey], to downbear lung counterflow. This is the subtlety of a circuitous and exhaustive systematic approach.

(4) Nevertheless, the dosage must not exceed a half square-*cùn* spoon full or it will result in diarrhea. [This would] cause lung qì to descend and drain out through the large intestine.

(5) [With this formula], you never have to worry about counterflow cough and ascent of qì again.

又方

半夏	二斤，去皮，河水洗六七度，完用
白礬	一斤，末之
丁香	各四兩，粗搗
甘草	
草豆蔻	
川升麻	
縮砂	

（一）上七味，以好酒一斗，與半夏拌和勻。

（二）同浸，春冬三七日，夏秋七日，密封口，日足取出。

（三）用冷水急洗，風吹乾。

（四）每服一粒，嚼破，用薑湯下。

（五）或乾吃，候六十日乾，方得服。

VI.3.d Another Formula

Ingredients

bànxià	1 *jīn*, peeled and rinsed in river water six or seven times, use whole.
báifán	1 *jīn*, pulverized
dīngxiāng	coarsely crushed, 4 *liǎng* each
gāncǎo	
cǎodòukòu	
chuānshēngmá	
suōshā	

Editorial comment: It is doubtful whether this is really Sūn Sīmiǎo's formula.

Preparation

(1) Of the seven ingredients above, use the *bànxià* to stir the others in 1 *dǒu* of high-quality liquor until everything is evenly combined.

(2) Soak everything together, in the spring and winter for three times seven days, in the summer and fall for seven days, [in a container] with a tightly sealed opening. When the days are complete, take it out.

(3) Use cold water to rinse it immediately and then let the wind blow it dry.

(4) Take 1 grain-sized piece per dose. Chew it to break it up and use ginger decoction to get it down.

(5) Alternatively, to eat it dry, wait until you have let it dry for 60 days, and only ingest it afterwards.

《衍義》

（一）前方用蜂蜜製杏仁以潤肺燥咳逆。

（二）此方用酒制半夏以逐胃濕痰氣，其自礬等
　　　味藉以解半夏之毒，並助胃健運之力耳。

Yǎn Yì (Expanded Meaning)

(1) The formula before the present one used the effect of honey-processed *xìngrén* to [treat] counterflow cough by moistening the lung dryness.

(2) The present formula uses the effect of liquor-processed *bànxià* to expel phlegm and damp qì from the stomach. It relies on the other ingredients, from *báifán* on, to resolve the toxicity of *bànxià* while at the same time supporting the stomach's strength to fortify and transport.

八味生薑煎

治少小嗽方。

生薑	七兩
乾薑	四兩
桂心	二兩
甘草	三兩
杏仁	一斤
款冬花	各三兩
紫菀	
蜜	一斤

（一）上合諸藥，末之，微火上煎取如飴餔。

（二）量其大小多少與兒含咽之，百日小兒如棗核許，日四五服，甚有驗。

八味生薑煎《衍義》

此治肺氣咳嗽氣逆。用蜂蜜者，藉以制姜、桂之燥也。

VI.3.e Bā Wèi Shēngjiāng Jiān (Eight-Ingredients Fresh Ginger Brew)

Indication

A formula to treat cough in children.

Ingredients

shēngjiāng	*7 liǎng*
gānjiāng	*4 liǎng*
guìxīn	*2 liǎng*
gāncǎo	*3 liǎng*
xìngrén	*1 jīn*
kuǎndōnghuā	*3 liǎng* each
zǐwǎn	
fēngmì	*1 jīn*

Preparation

(1) Combine the various herbs above and pulverize them. Simmer them [with the honey] over a small flame until reduced to the consistency of malt candy or mush.

(2) Measure out an amount in accordance with the child's age and give it to the child to hold in the mouth and throat. For a small child a hundred days old, give an amount roughly the size of a jujube pit, 4-5 doses a day. [This formula] has great efficacy.

Bā Wèi Shēngjiāng Jiān (Eight-Ingredients Fresh Ginger Brew) *Yǎn Yì* **Expanded Meaning**

This formula treats lung qì cough and qì counterflow. It includes honey because it relies on it to restrain the dryness of the [dried and fresh] ginger and *guìzhī*.

四物款冬丸

治小兒嗽，日中瘥，夜甚，初不得息，不能複啼
方。

款冬花	各一兩半
紫菀	
桂心	半兩
伏龍肝	六銖

上，末之，蜜和如泥，取如棗核大敷乳頭，令兒
飲之，日三敷之，漸漸令兒飲之。

四物款冬丸《衍義》

（一）咳嗽晝愈夜甚，在少年當責之陰虛，在老
人當責之血燥，在小兒當責肺胃虛冷。

（二）故用桂心、伏龍肝之辛溫實脾，以助款
冬、紫菀溫肺之力。

VI.3.f Sì Wù Kuǎndōng Wán (Four-Ingredient Coltsfoot Pill)

Indication

A formula for small children, to treat cough that improves during the day but worsens at night. At the onset [of coughing], the patient is unable to breathe and is unable to cry repeatedly.

Ingredients

kuǎndōnghuā	1.5 *liǎng* each
zǐwǎn	
guìxīn	0.5 *liǎng*
fúlónggān	6 *zhū*

Preparation

Pulverize the ingredients above and mix with honey into a mud-like consistency. Take an amount the size of a jujube pit and apply it to the nipple of the [mother's] breast. Have the child nurse there. Apply it three times a day and little by little have the child drink it down.

Sì Wù Kuǎndōng Wán (Four-Ingredient Coltsfoot Pill) *Yǎn Yì* **(Expanded Meaning)**

(1) A cough that improves during the day and worsens at night must be blamed on yīn vacuity when it occurs in childhood, and on blood dryness when it occurs in old patients. In small children, it must be blamed on vacuity cold in the lung and stomach.

(2) Therefore we use the acridity and warmth of *guìxīn* and *fúlónggān* to make the spleen replete, thereby assisting the power of *kuǎndōnghuā* and *zǐwǎn* to warm the lung.

菖蒲丸

治小兒暴冷嗽，及積風冷嗽，兼氣逆鳴方。

菖蒲	
烏頭	
杏仁	
礬石	各六銖
細辛	
皂莢	
款冬花	
乾薑	
桂心	各十八銖
紫菀	
蜀椒	五合
吳茱萸	六合

VI.3.g Chāngpú Wán (Acorus Pill)

Indication

A formula for small children, to treat coughs of the fulminant cold [type] as well as coughs of the accumulated wind and cold [type], concurrent with qì counterflow and making sounds.[9]

Ingredients

chāngpú	
wūtóu	
xìngrén	6 *zhū* each
fánshí	
xìxīn	
zàojiá	
kuǎndōnghuā	
gānjiāng	18 *zhū* each
guìxīn	
zǐwǎn	
shǔjiāo	5 *gě**
wúzhūyú	6 *gě*

Translator's Note: Some editions, including the *Yǎn Yì* edition, have 5 *zhū* instead.

---

9   鳴 *míng* literally refers to the sounds made by birds. In most medical contexts, it either denotes intestinal rumbling (腸鳴 *cháng míng*) or ringing in the ears (耳鳴 *ěr míng*). In the present context, it most likely just means sounds emitted by the patient. Grammatically, it is also possible to read 氣逆鳴 as a compound, and I leave it to the reader to contemplate what "qì counterflow sounds" might sound like.

（一）上十二味，末之，蜜丸如梧子。

（二）三歲兒飲服五丸，加至十丸，日三。

（三）兒小以意減之，兒大以意加之，暴嗽數服便瘥。

菖蒲丸《衍義》

（一）《本經》以菖蒲為風寒濕痹、欬逆上氣要藥。

（二）世人但知其通心利竅、明耳目，出聲之功，欬逆絕不知用。

（三）是慮其溫燥也。

（四）其辛、烏、姜、桂、椒、茰，總取其辛溫散冷之用。

Preparation

(1) Pulverize the twelve ingredients above and process into honey pills the size of *wútóng* seeds.

(2) For a child of 3 *suì*, give 5 pills per dose in liquid, increasing the dose to up to 10 pills, 3 times a day.

(3) For younger children, decrease the dosage at your discretion. For older children, increase the dosage at your discretion. For fulminant cough, give frequent doses, and [the patient] will recover.

Chāngpú Wán (Acorus Pill) *Yǎn Yì* (Expanded Meaning)

(1) The *Shénnóng Běncǎo Jīng* describes *chāngpú* as an essential medicinal for wind-, cold-, and damp-related bì impediment, cough with counterflow, and ascent of qì.

(2) The common people are only aware of its achievements in opening up the flow[10] in the heart and disinhibiting the orifices, sharpening the ears and eyes, and emitting sound. They are utterly unaware of its use for cough with counterflow.

(3) This [latter medicinal effect of *chāngpú* can be known when we] consider its warming and drying [nature].

(4) The *xìxīn, wūtóu, gānjiāng, guìxīn, shǔjiāo*, and *wúzhūyú* [in this formula] are all included because of their acrid and warm cold-dissipating effect.

---

10 See Commentary VI.3.g by Sabine Wilms

（五）其妙尤在稀涎散之皂莢、礬石助菖蒲開竅
滌痰之力。

（六）杏仁、款冬、紫菀不過藉以引諸藥入肺經
耳。

Commentary VI.3.g ◂ Sabine Wilms

通心 *tōng xīn*: The Practical Dictionary of Chinese Medicine translates 通 in most medical contexts as "to free," as for example in the compounds 通耳 "to free the ears" or 通經 "to free the menses." I could have just translated the compound here as "to free the heart" and left it to the reader to figure out what that means. But on the one hand, the potential for a misunderstanding is too great, and on the other, the character 通 has a very specific meaning that is not fully conveyed by that English translation. Defined in the *Shuōwén Jiězì* as 達 *dá* (to arrive [at a destination]), 通 carries the connotation of restoring healthy flow and "reaching" in the sense of opening up interaction with the outside, reflected in the modern compound 交通 *jiāotōng* meaning "traffic" or "communications." One way to visualize it is in the action of restoring the free flow through a blocked straw or bamboo tube by vigorously blowing through it or poking a hole through the obstruction. In the present context, 通心 can perhaps be rendered most literally as "restoring the unobstructed flow or movement in or to and from the heart." One way that we can interpret this meaning would be as "to open up communication in the heart" but it could also refer on a more physiological level to unblocking the orifices of the heart.

(5) The [present treatment's] subtlety lies specifically in [its use of] *zàojiá* and *fánshí*, which make up Xī Xián Sǎn[11] to assist the force of *chāngpú* to open the orifices and flush out phlegm.

(6) *Xìngrén, kuǎndōnghuā,* and *zǐwǎn* are included here merely for the purpose of drawing the other ingredients into the lung channel.

---

11 I read the three characters 稀涎散 as a reference to a formula of this name (lit. "Drool-Thinning Powder, also known as Bèi Jí Xī Xián Sǎn 備急稀涎散, "Emergency-Preparedness Drool-Thinning Powder"), which is made up of the two ingredients *zàojiá* and *fánshí*. The earliest evidence of this formula I have been able to find is in the Sòng dynasty text *Shèng Jì Zǒng Lù*. An alternative reading of the line, which is suggested by the way the modern editors of the *Yǎn Yì* edition have punctuated, placing a period between this phrase and the next, would be: "The subtlety lies specifically in its ability to thin drool and disperse it." Given the fact that this characteristic would apply better to the following two medicinals, *zàojiá* and *fánshí*, however, this punctuation makes less sense to me.

Commentary VI.3.g ✦ Julian Scott

I think this refers to what we would call croup. I am not sure how the character for drool could be translated, but in croup, the main thing is to soften the hard mucus. It can then be expectorated, or even passed out through the stools. From a clinical point of view, when looking at the tongue, one can see the saliva (presumably the drool) as very thick and tenuous when the cough is harsh, and much more runny when the cough becomes productive.

桂枝湯

治少小十日以上至五十日，卒得警咳，吐乳，嘔逆，暴嗽，晝夜不得息方。

桂枝	半兩
甘草	二兩半
紫菀	十八銖
麥門冬	一兩十八銖

上四味，咬咀，以水二升，煮取半升，以綿著湯中，捉綿滴兒口中，晝夜四五過與之。

節乳哺。

VI.4 Modifications of *Shāng Hán Lùn* Formulas

VI.4.a Guìzhī Tāng (Cinnamon Twig Decoction)

Indication
A formula for children from ten to fifty days after birth, to treat sudden contraction of a sonorous cough with vomiting of breast milk, retching counterflow, fulminant cough, and no rest [from the condition] day or night.

Ingredients

guìzhī	0.5 *liǎng*
gāncǎo	2.5 *liǎng*
zǐwǎn	18 *zhū*
màiméndōng	1 *liǎng* and 18 *zhū*

Preparation
Pound the four ingredients above and decoct in 2 *shēng* of water until reduced to 0.5 *shēng*. Place silk floss in the decoction and then take it out [and use it] to drip [some of the medicine] into the child's mouth. Administer [the medicine] four or five times throughout the day and night.

Moderate nursing and feeding.

麻黃湯

治少小卒肩息上氣，不得安，此惡風入肺方。

麻黃	一兩
甘草	一兩
桂心	五寸
五味子	半斤
半夏	各二兩
生薑	

（一）上六味，咬咀，以水五升，煮取二升。

（二）百日兒服一合，大小節度服之，便愈。

VI.4.b Máhuáng Tāng (Ephedra Decoction)

Indication

A formula for children, to treat sudden [raised-]shoulder breathing, qì ascent, and inability to be at ease. This is malign wind entering the lung.

Ingredients

máhuáng	1 *liǎng*
gāncǎo	1 *liǎng*
guìxīn	5 *cùn*
wǔwèizǐ	0.5 *jīn*
bànxià	2 *liǎng* each
shēngjiāng	

Preparation

(1) Pound the six ingredients above and decoct in 5 *shēng* of water until reduced to 2 *shēng*.

(2) For a hundred-day-old child, give 1 *gě* per dose. Adjust the dosage in accordance with the child's age. Recovery will ensue.

Commentary VI.4.b ✦ Julian Scott

I think this refers to cough-induced asthma. In infants this is usually due to Lung and Kidney weakness hence the strong tonics.

《衍義》

（一）桂枝湯，風傷衛藥也。

（二）以本方無治馨咳藥，故去芍藥、姜、棗，而易紫菀、門冬。

（三）引領桂枝、甘草，以開發肺胃逆氣。

（四）麻黃湯，寒傷營藥也。

（五）以本方無治肩息藥，故藉小青龍去白芍、細辛，易生薑以辟除惡風痰氣。

（六）皆長沙方中變法。豈特嬰兒主治哉。

Yǎn Yì (Expanded Meaning)

(1) Guìzhī Tāng is a medicine for wind damaging the *wèi* defense level.

(2) Because the root formula[12] does not contain medicinals that treat sonorous coughing, [the present formula] has removed *sháoyào*, *shēngjiāng*, and *dàzǎo*, and substituted *zǐwǎn* and *màiméndōng* in their place

(3) It draws on the leadership of *guìzhī* and *gāncǎo* to open and effuse the counterflow qì in the lung and stomach.

(4) Máhuáng Tāng is a medicine for cold damaging the *yíng* provisioning level.

(5) Since the root formula[13] does not contain medicinals that treat [raised-]shoulder breathing, [the present formula] also relies on [ingredients from] Xiǎoqīnglóng Tāng, but without *báisháo* and *xìxīn* and substituting *shēngjiāng* to expel phlegm qì from malign wind.

(6) Both of these formulas are modifications of formulas from Chángshā.[14] How could these formulas possibly be indicated specifically for infants alone!

---

12 This is a reference to the standard formula for Guìzhī Tāng from the *Shāng Hán Lùn*, which resolves the exterior, dispels wind, and harmonizes *yíng* provisioning and *wèi* defense in exterior vacuity conditions with spontaneous sweating.

13 This is a reference to the standard formula for Máhuáng Tāng from the *Shāng Hán Lùn*, which treats externally contracted wind-cold conditions with exterior repletion, resolving the exterior by promoting sweating, diffusing the lung, and stabilizing panting.

14 A reference to Zhāng Zhòngjǐng's classic formulas from the *Shāng Hán Lùn*.

CHAPTER SEVEN: AGGREGATIONS, BINDS, Distension, AND FULLNESS

癖結脹滿第七

(35 formulas, 1 moxibustion method)

紫雙丸

（一）治小兒身熱頭痛，食飲不消，腹中脹滿；
　　　或小腹絞痛，大小便不利；或重下數起；
　　　小兒無異疾，惟飲食過度，不知自止，哺
　　　乳失節；或驚悸寒熱。惟此丸治之。不
　　　瘥，更可重服。

（二）小兒欲下，是其蒸候；哺食減少，氣息不
　　　快，夜啼不眠，是腹內不調，悉宜用此
　　　丸，不用他藥。數用神驗。

（三）千金不傳方。

Commentary VII.1.a ✠ Julian Scott

This is a condition that we might call 'full heat in the stomach with empty spleen'. The heat leads to excessive appetite and overeating, which in turn leads to food accumulating in the abdomen. This decays and causes further heat which, rises up to the stomach. It is not infrequent in the practice.

VII.1 Digestive Issues in Newborns

VII.1.a Zǐ Shuāng Wán (Purple Paired Pill)

Indication

(1) A treatment for small children [who are suffering from] generalized heat and headache, failure to disperse food and drink, and Distension and fullness in the abdomen, possibly with wringing pain in the lesser abdomen and inhibited defecation and urination, or with repeatedly occurring severe bowel movements.[1] [Also a treatment] for small children who have no other illness but who only eat or drink too much, do not know when to stop, and feed and nurse without moderation, possibly with fright palpitations and cold [effusion and aversion to] heat. [Giving] these pills alone will treat [such patients]. If [the patient] is not cured, you can give another dose.[2]

continued on next page

---

1 重下數起 *zhòng xià shuò qǐ*: An alternative interpretation would be to read 重 not as *zhòng* (meaning "heavy, severe, serious") but as *chóng*, meaning "double" or "repeated," in which case it would merely reinforce the meaning of 數起 ("repeatedly / frequently occurring").

2 更可重服 *gèng kě chóng fú*: Read literally, this phrase translates as "You may further give a double dose." It is possible to interpret this as recommending that the patient is given a second dose that is twice the amount of the first treatment, if the first treatment is ineffective. Given the strength of the formula and the fragile nature of small children, however, I interpret it as stating that it is safe to give a second dose of a pair of pills, if the first dose does not do the trick. To complicate matters further, it is also possible to read the last two sentences as a single sentence: "If you treat these [conditions] only by means of these pills and there is no cure, you can give another [double] dose."

EDITORIAL NOTE:

（一）臣億等詳序例中凡云服紫丸者即前變蒸篇十四
　　　味者是也。

（二）云服紫丸不下者，服赤丸，赤丸瘥快，病重者
　　　當用之。

（三）方中並無赤丸，而此用朱砂，又力緊於紫丸，
　　　疑此即赤丸也。

(1) Whenever instructions in the detailed arrangements
by your servant Yì[3] and his collaborators call for
taking "Purple Pills" (Zǐ Wán 紫丸), this refers to the
[formula with that name that has] fourteen ingredients, listed above in the chapter on Steamings and
Transformations.[4]

(2) As stated there, "if the patient has taken Purple Pills
and these have failed to induce a bowel movement, he
or she should take 'Red Pills' (Chì Wán 赤丸). Recovery with Red Pills is fast, and if the condition is serious,
you must use them."

(3) Among the formulas [in the *Qiān Jīn Fāng*], there is no
[formula for] Red Pills to be found. Nevertheless, the
formula above uses *zhūshā*, and in addition its strength
is more urgent than Purple Pills, so we wonder if this
formula here is not identical with these Red Pills.

3　臣億 Chén Yì: Literally "your servant Yì," this is a reference by Lín
Yì 林億, the editor in charge of the Sòng dynasty revision of the *Qiān Jīn
Fāng*, to himself.

4　See "Venerating the Root, Part One," chapter 1, "Preface," pp. 33 ff for
the formula for "Purple Pills."

(2) If small children are about to have bowel movements, these are the symptoms of their "steaming."[5] If they [additionally suffer from] reduced food intake, belabored breathing, and crying at night instead of sleeping, they are the symptoms of a lack of attunement in the abdomen. [In that case,] it is entirely appropriate to use these pills. Do not use any other medicine. Repeatedly using this medicine is divinely effective.

(3) A formula not to be passed on [even] for a thousand [pieces of] gold[6]:

---

5   My best guess for the meaning of the first phrase 小兒欲下 *xiǎo ér yù xià* ("if small children are about to have bowel movements") is that this refers to babies who do not suffer from continued constipation but have regular healthy bowel movements when they exhibit some or all of the other symptoms described above. For the significance of "steaming," see Chapter One on this key stage of neonatal development. As a whole, this sentence thus means that the above-listed symptoms, when experienced by infants with healthy bowel movements, characterize merely a normal physiological stage of neonatal development, but need to be managed more actively by medical intervention when they are accompanied by reduced food intake, belabored breathing, and crying at night.

6   千金不傳方 *qiān jīn bù chuán fāng*: This phrase presents a bit of a difficulty for our contemporary way of thinking about medicine, because it seems to blatantly contradict Sūn Sīmiǎo's commitment to nurturing and preserving life by transmitting and sharing vital medical information for the greater benefit of humanity. My best guess is that Sūn Sīmiǎo copied formulas in their entirety and therefore preserved the wording of this formula literally. And in the cultural context of professional medical practice in medieval China, a statement such as this makes perfect sense, signifying that this formula was so eminently valuable that no doctor would ever sell it, even for a thousand pieces of gold. Jealous protection of the secrets of one's trade and transmission only to a small circle of select descendants or disciples has been a hallmark of professional medical practice throughout the history of Chinese medicine.

巴豆	十八銖
麥門冬	十銖
甘草	五銖
甘遂	二銖
朱砂	二銖
蠟	十銖
蕤核仁	十八銖
牡蠣	八銖

（一）上八味，以湯熟洗巴豆，研，新布絞去油。別搗甘草、甘遂、牡蠣、麥門冬，下篩訖。研蕤核仁令極熟，乃納散更搗二千杵。

（二）藥燥不能相丸，更入少蜜足之。

Ingredients

bādòu	18 *zhū*
màiméndōng	10 *zhū*
gāncǎo	5 *zhū*
gānsuì	2 *zhū*
zhūshā	2 *zhū*
fēnglà	10 *zhū*
ruíhérén	18 *zhū*
mǔlì	8 *zhū*

Preparation

(1) Of the eight ingredients above, thoroughly rinse the *bādòu* in hot water, grind, and then wring them out in new cloth to remove the oil. Separately pound the *gāncǎo*, *gānsuì*, *mǔlì*, and *màiméndōng* and sift them all the way down. Grind the *ruíhérén* until extremely fine and add to the powder. Pound again for two thousand times.

(2) If the medicine is too dry to shape into pills, add a little honey, just until it is enough.

（三）半歲兒服如荏子一雙；一歲、二歲兒服如半麻子一雙；三四歲者服如麻子二丸；五六歲者服如大麻子二丸；七歲、八歲服如小豆二丸；九歲、十歲微大於小豆二丸。

（四）常以雞鳴時服，至日出時不下者，熱粥飲數合即下。

（五）丸皆雙出也。下甚者，飲以冷粥即止。

(3) For a child half a *suì* old, give a pair [of the pills] the size of perilla seeds.[7] For a child of one to two *suì*, give a pair the size of half a hemp seed. For a child of three to four *suì*, give two pills the size of hemp seeds. For a child of five to six *suì*, give two pills the size of cannabis seeds. For a child of seven to eight *suì*, give two pills the size of mung beans. For a child of nine to ten *suì*, give two pills that are slightly larger than mung beans.

(4) Always [have the patient] take [the medicine] at the time of the [first] rooster crow. If [the medicine] has failed to induce a bowel movement by sunrise, having the patient drink several *gě* of hot gruel will immediately cause it.

(5) The pills all emerge in pairs. If the downward-moving [effect of the medicine] is too strong, having the patient drink cold gruel will stop [the medicine's action].

---

7   荏: *Rěn* is a character referring to the plant that is now more commonly referred to as 白蘇 *bái sū* (Perilla Alba). I read the expression "one pair" (一雙 *yī shuāng*) literally, to mean that the patient should take two pills the size of tiny perilla seeds. Given the young age, these instructions make perfect sense.

紫雙丸《衍義》

（一）小兒無異疾，惟飲食之過度，故宜巴豆之辛散，兼甘遂之苦寒，以蕩滌癖積。

（二）蕤仁除心腹邪熱結氣；麥冬治腸中傷飽，胃絡脈絕，羸瘦短氣。

（三）牡蠣散內結積，蜂蠟清胃，甘草和中，丹砂安神，不使巴豆、甘遂侵犯正氣也。

Zǐ Shuāng Wán (Purple Paired Pill) *Yǎn Yì* (Expanded Meaning)

(1) For small children who have no other illness but who only eat or drink too much, it is indeed appropriate to combine the acrid dissipating [action] of *bādòu* with the bitter and cold [nature] of *gānsuì*, to flush out the aggregations and gatherings.

(2) *Ruíhérén* eliminates the evil heat and bound qì in the heart and abdomen. *Màiméndōng* treats damage from overeating in the intestines, interruption of network vessels and channels in the stomach, and marked emaciation with shortness of breath.

(3) *Mǔlì* dissipates internal binds and gatherings, *fēnglà* clears the stomach, *gāncǎo* harmonizes the center, and *dānshā* sets the spirit at ease. This prevents *bādòu* and *gānsuì* from infringing on right qì.

治小兒胎中宿熱，乳母飲食粗惡辛苦，乳汁不起兒，乳哺不為肌膚，心腹痞滿，萎黃瘦瘠，四肢痿躄繚戾，服之可令充悅方。

芍藥	二兩半
大黃	一兩
甘草	半兩
柴胡	二兩
鱉甲	一兩半
茯苓各	
乾薑	半兩*
人參	一兩

Commentary VII.1.b ❧ Julian Scott

In the West, the most common cause of this condition is immunization.

VII.1.b Formula for Abiding Heat

Indication

A formula for small children, to treat abiding heat [that was contracted] in utero, [the effects of] the wet nurse or mother eating or drinking poor-quality,[8] acrid, or bitter substances, failure of the breast milk to sustain the child,[9] feeding or nursing without producing flesh and skin, *pǐ* glomus and fullness in the heart and abdomen, withering jaundice and marked emaciation, and crippling wilt and hypertonicity in the four limbs. Taking this formula will cause the child to fill out and be happy.

Ingredients

sháoyào	2.5 *liǎng*
dàhuáng	1 *liǎng*
gāncǎo	0.5 *liǎng*
cháihú	2 *liǎng*
biējiǎ	1.5 *liǎng* each
fúlíng	
*gānjiāng**	0.5 *liǎng*
rénshēn	1 *liǎng*

*Editorial comment: If there is heat, substitute *zhǐshí* instead.

---

8 粗惡 *cū è*: Literally, these two characters means "coarse" or "rough" and "distasteful," "malign," or even "nauseating," respectively. As a compound, the expression refers to low quality, lack of refinement, or unwholesomeness, as associated with poverty and/or care in preparation. The concrete meaning of this phrase in our modern times is obviously different from what it meant in medieval China, when it referred to rotten or dirty food or to a diet of poverty devoid of meat and other vital nutritious substances. In direct contrast, our modern diet seems to be suffering from the exact opposite, namely an excess of refinement and lack of foods in their natural, unadulterated state. In any case, the formula is indicated for babies who are suffering from the effects of consuming breast milk from a mother with an inappropriate or inadequate diet. By extension, it is easy to see how this formula can also be applied to babies fed on formula or milk from animal sources.

9 In an interesting textual variation, the *Sūn Zhēn Rén* edition has here 乳汁不下 ("failure of the breast milk to descend") instead of 乳汁不起兒. Below, the phrase 心腹痞滿 ("*pǐ* glomus and fullness in the heart and abdomen") is replaced by 心腹不滿 ("lack of fullness in the heart and abdomen") in this same edition.

（一）上八味，末之，蜜丸如大豆。

（二）服一丸，一歲以上乳服三丸，七歲兒服十
　　　丸，日二。

《衍義》

（一）嬰兒胎稟中有宿熱，故取小柴胡以和之。

（二）以半夏之辛燥，故易茯苓；黃芩苦寒，故
　　　易鱉甲；生薑辛散，故易乾姜。

（三）其芍藥、大黃乃大柴胡中主藥。

（四）去大棗，不去人參、甘草者，惡其膩膈，
　　　取其安中也。

Preparation

(1) Pulverize the eight ingredients above and form into honey pills the size of soybeans.

(2) Give one pill per dose. For a child of more than one *suì*, give three pills per dose in breast milk. For a child of seven *suì*, give ten pills per dose. Give two doses a day.

Yǎn Yì (Expanded Meaning)

(1) Because the infants [for whom this formula is indicated] are suffering from the presence of abiding heat that they received while still in utero, we choose Xiǎo Cháihú Tāng to harmonize them.

(2) Because of the acrid and drying nature of *bànxià*, [the present formula] substitutes *fúlíng*. Because of the bitter and cold nature of *huángqín*, [the present formula] substitutes *biējiǎ*. Because of the acrid and dissipating nature of *shēngjiāng*, [the present formula] substitutes *gānjiāng*.

(3) The *sháoyào* and *dàhuáng* in the present formula are the ruling medicinals in Dà Cháihú Tāng.

(4) The reason why [the present formula] has removed *dàzǎo* but not *rénshēn* and *gāncǎo* is that [the former ingredient's] stickiness in the diaphragm is bad while [the latter ingredients] have been chosen [for their ability to] set the center at ease.

牛黃丸

治小兒宿乳不消，腹痛驚啼方。

牛黃	三銖
附子	二枚
真珠	一兩
巴豆	一兩
杏仁	一兩

（一）上五味，搗附子、真珠，末之，下篩。

（二）別搗巴豆、杏仁令如泥，納藥及牛黃，搗一千二百杵，藥成。

（三）若乾，入少蜜足之。

（四）百日兒服如粟米一丸，三歲兒服如麻子一丸，五六歲兒服如胡豆一丸。

VII.2 Formulas for Resolving Abiding Food, Heat, and Phlegm

VII.2.a Niúhuáng Wán (Bovine Bezoar Pill)

Indication

A formula for small children, to treat abiding breast milk that is failing to disperse, with abdominal pain, fright, and crying.

Ingredients

niúhuáng	3 *zhū*
fùzǐ	2 pieces
zhēnzhū	1 *liǎng*
bādòu	1 *liǎng*
xìngrén	1 *liǎng*

Preparation

(1) Of the five ingredients above, pound the *fùzǐ* and *zhēnzhū*, and pulverize and sift them.

(2) Separately pound the *bādòu* and *xìngrén*, processing them into a mud-like consistency. Add the herbs and the *niúhuáng*, and pound [everything] another 1200 times. [With this,] the medicine is completed.

(3) If it is dry, add a little honey just until it is enough.

(4) For a child a hundred days old, give one pill about the size of a millet grain per dose. For a child of three *suì*, give one pill the size of a hemp seed per dose. For a child five or six *suì* old, give one pill the size of a fava bean per dose.

（五）日二，先乳哺了服之。

（六）膈上下悉當微轉。

（七）藥完出者病愈。散出者更服，以藥完出為
度。

芒硝紫丸

治小兒宿食、癖氣、痰飲，往來寒熱，不欲食，
消瘦方。

芒硝	各四兩
大黃	
半夏	二兩
代赭	一兩
甘遂	二兩
巴豆	二百枚
杏仁	一百二十枚

（一）上七味，末之。　　別搗巴豆、杏仁，治如
膏。

(5) Twice a day, give a dose before nursing or feeding.

(6) [In the area] all above and below the diaphragm, there should be a slight turning [sensation].

(7) If the medicine comes out in its entirety, the disease is cured. If only scattered pieces [of the medicine] come out, give another dose. Take the fact that the medicine has come out in its entirety as your measure [that you can stop taking more doses].

VII.2.b Mángxiāo Zǐ Wán (Mirabilite Purple Pill)

Indication

A formula for small children to treat abiding food, qì aggregations, and phlegm rheum, with alternating heat [effusion] and [aversion to] cold, lack of appetite,[10] and emaciation.

Ingredients

mángxiāo	4 *liǎng* each
dàhuáng	
bànxià	2 *liǎng*
dàizhǐ	1 *liǎng*
gānsuì	2 *liǎng*
bādòu	200 pieces
xìngrén	120 pieces

Preparation

(1) Of the seven ingredients above, pulverize [the first five]. Separately pound the *bādòu* and *xìngrén*, processing them into a paste-like consistency.

---

10 An alternate version of this line instead has 不飲食 *bù yǐn shí* ("not drinking and eating") instead of 不欲食 *bú yù shí* ("not wanting to eat").

（二）旋納藥末，搗三千杵，令相和合，強者納
少蜜。

（三）百日兒服如胡豆一丸，過百日至一歲服二
丸，隨兒大小，以意節度。

（四）當候兒大便中藥出為愈。若不出，更服如
初。

Commentary VII.2b,c ❧ Julian Scott

When a child has a lot of phlegm accumulation in the abdomen, it gives rise to periodic symptoms. e.g. the appetite may be voracious one day, and poor for the next few days. The explanation for this is that eating food 'stirs up' phlegm, which then rises up to the stomach making the child nauseous (sometimes they even vomit phlegm). After a few days of near fasting, the Spleen manages to transform the phlegm so the stomach is ready to take more food. One may see alternating hot and cold symptoms going with this.

(2) With a rotating motion, add the pulverized herbs and pound [everything] with a pestle three thousand times until thoroughly mixed. If it is stiff, add a little honey.

(3) For a child of a hundred days, give one pill roughly the size of a fava bean per dose. For a child between a hundred days and one *suì*, give two pills. Measure the amount at your discretion in accordance with the child's age.

(4) You must wait until the medicine comes out in the child's stool, which means recovery. If it does not come out, give another dose like in the beginning.

治八歲以上兒，熱結痰實，不能食，自下方。

芍藥	各二兩
梔子	
柴胡	一兩六銖
升麻	各二兩半
黃連	
黃芩	
竹葉，切	一升半
桔梗	一兩半
細辛	十五銖
知母	各二兩
大黃	

（一）上十一味，㕮咀，以水六升，煮取一升八
合，去滓。

（二）分四服，十歲兒為三服。

VII.2.c Unnamed Formula

Indication

A formula for children above the age of eight *suì*, to treat heat bind and phlegm repletion with inability to eat and spontaneous bowel movements.

Ingredients

sháoyào	2 *liǎng* each
zhīzhǐ	
cháihú	1 *liǎng* 6 *zhū*
shēngmá	2.5 *liǎng* each
huánglián	
huángqín	
zhúyè, chopped	1.5 *shēng*
jiégěng	1.5 *liǎng*
xìxīn	15 *zhū*
zhīmǔ	2 *liǎng* each
dàhuáng	

Preparation

(1) Pound the eleven ingredients above and decoct in 6 *shēng* of water until reduced to 1 *shēng* and 8 *gě*. Remove the dregs.

(2) Divide into four doses. For a child of ten *suì*, divide it into three doses.[11]

---

11 Editorial note: Another edition includes 1.5 *liǎng* each of *zhǐshí* and *xìngrén* but does not contain *jiégěng* or *huánglián*.

治十五以下兒，熱結多痰，食飲減，自下方。

大黃	各三兩
柴胡	
黃芩	
枳實	一兩十八銖
升麻	各二兩半
芍藥	
知母	
梔子	
生薑	十八銖
杏仁	二兩
竹葉，切	一升半

（一）上十一味，咬咀，以水六升半，煮取二升。

（二）十歲至十五，分三服。

VII.2.d Unnamed Formula

Indication

A formula for children under the age of fifteen *suì*, to treat heat bind and profuse phlegm with reduced eating and drinking and spontaneous bowel movements.

Ingredients

dàhuáng	3 *liǎng* each
cháihú	
huángqín	
zhǐshí	1 *liǎng*, 18 *zhū*
shēngmá	2.5 *liǎng* each
sháoyào	
zhīmǔ	
zhīzhǐ	
shēngjiāng	18 *zhū*
xìngrén	2 *liǎng*
zhúyè, chopped	1.5 *shēng*

Preparation

(1) Pound the eleven ingredients above and decoct in 6.5 *shēng* of water until reduced to 2 *shēng*.

(2) For a child of ten to fifteen *suì*, divide into three doses.

牛黃雙丸

治小兒結實，乳食不消，心腹痛方。

牛黃	各半兩
太山甘遂	
真珠	六銖
杏仁	各一兩
芍藥	
黃芩	
巴豆	十八銖

（一）上七味，末之，蜜丸。

（二）一歲兒飲服如麻子二丸，但隨兒大小加減
之。

VII.2.e Niúhuáng Shuāng Wán (Bovine Bezoar Paired Pill)

Indication

A formula for small children, to treat binding and repletion, failure to disperse breast milk and food, and heart and abdominal pain.

Ingredients

niúhuáng	0.5 *liǎng* each
tàishāngānsuì	
zhēnzhū	6 *zhū*
xìngrén	1 *liǎng* each
sháoyào	
huángqín	
bādòu	18 *zhū*

Preparation

(1) Pulverize the seven ingredients above and [process them into] honey pills.

(2) For a child of one *suì*, give 2 pills the size of hemp seeds in liquid. Simply increase or decrease the amount in accordance with the child's age.

牛黃鱉甲丸

治少小癖實壯熱，食不消化，中惡忤氣方。

牛黃	半兩
鱉甲	
麥曲	
柴胡	
大黃	各一兩
枳實	
芎藭	
厚朴	
茯苓	
桂心	各半兩
芍藥	
乾薑	

（一）上十二味，末之，蜜丸如小豆大。

（二）日三服，以意量之。

VII.2.f Niúhuáng Biējiǎ Wán (Bovine Bezoar and Turtle Shell Pill)

Indication

A formula for children, to treat aggregations and repletion with vigorous heat [effusion], failure to transform food, and malignity strike and [intrusive] upset qì.[12]

Ingredients

niúhuáng	0.5 *liǎng*
biējiǎ	
màiqū	
cháihú	
dàhuáng	1 *liǎng* each
zhǐshí	
xiōngqióng	
hòupò	
fúlíng	
guìxīn	0.5 *liǎng* each
sháoyào	
gānjiāng	

Preparation

(1) Pulverize the twelve ingredients above and [process into] honey pills about the size of mung beans.

(2) Give three doses per day, measuring it at your discretion.

---

12   For more information on this condition, see *Venerating the Root, Part One,* chapter four on "Intrusive Upset," specifically pp. 235-237.

芫花丸

治小兒心下痞，痰癖結聚，腹大脹滿，身體壯熱，不欲哺乳方。

芫花	一兩
大黃	
雄黃	各二兩半
黃芩	一兩

（一）上四味，末之，蜜和，更搗一千杵。

（二）三歲兒至一歲以下服如粟米一丸。

（三）欲服丸，納兒喉中，令母與乳。

（四）若長服消病者，當以意消息與服之，與乳哺相避。

VII.2.g Yuánhuā Wán (Genkwa Pill)

Indication

A formula for small children, to treat *pǐ* glomus below the heart, phlegm aggregations, and binds and gatherings, with abdominal enlargement, Distension, and fullness, vigorous generalized heat [effusion], and not wanting to feed or nurse.

Ingredients

yuánhuā	1 *liǎng*
dàhuáng	2.5 *liǎng* each
xiónghuáng	
huángqín	1 *liǎng*

Preparation

(1) Pulverize the four ingredients above. Combine with honey and pound again with a pestle a thousand times.

(2) For a child from three *suì* to under the age of one *suì*, give one pill the size of a millet grain per dose.

(3) When you want to give the pill, place it in the child's throat and have the mother breastfeed the child.

(4) If you are giving [the medicine] for an extended period of time and to dispel the illness, you must stop dispelling and then resume taking it at your discretion, spacing out doses in between nursing and feeding.

真珠丸

治小兒痰實結聚，宿癖，羸露，不能飲食方。

真珠	半兩
麥門冬	一兩
蕘仁	二百枚
巴豆	四十枚

（一）上四味，末之，蜜丸。

（二）期歲兒服二丸如小豆大，二百日兒服如麻子二丸。

（三）漸增，以知為度。

（四）當下病赤黃白黑葵汁，下勿絕藥，病盡下自止。

（五）久服使小兒肥白，已試驗。

VII.2.h Zhēnzhū Wán (Pearl Pill)

Indication

A formula for small children, to treat phlegm repletion, binds and gatherings, and abiding aggregations, with emaciation down to the bones and inability to eat and drink.

Ingredients

zhēnzhū	0.5 *liǎng*
màiméndōng	1 *liǎng*
ruíhérén	200 pieces
bādòu	40 pieces

Preparation

(1) Pulverize the four ingredients above and [process into] honey pills.

(2) For a child who has completed the first full year of life, the dose is 2 pills the size of mung beans. For a child of two hundred days, the dose is 2 pills the size of hemp seeds.

(3) Gradually increase the dosage, measuring it by when you notice an effect.

(4) You must expel the disease downward in the form of a red, yellow, white, or black liquid like mallow juice. When this downward expulsion occurs, do not interrupt taking the medicine! Once the disease has been expelled in its entirety, [the downward-expelling effect of the medicine] will stop on its own.

(5) Taking [this formula] for a long time makes small children chubby and white. Its efficacy is tested and verified.

鱉甲丸

治少小腹中結堅，脅下有疹，手足煩熱方。

鱉甲	
芍藥	各三十銖
大黃	
茯苓	
柴胡	各二十四銖
乾薑	
桂心	六銖
䗪蟲	各二十枚
蟒蛴	

（一）上九味，末之，蜜和。

（二）服如梧子七丸，漸漸加之，以知為度。

VII.2.i Biějiǎ Wán (Turtle Shell Pill)

Indication

A formula for children, to treat binding and hardening in the abdomen [that manifests] with the presence of papules below the rib-sides and vexing heat in the hands and feet.

Ingredients

biějiǎ	30 *zhū* each
sháoyào	
dàhuáng	
fúlíng	24 *zhū* each
cháihú	
gānjiāng,	
guìxīn,	6 *zhū*
zhèchóng	20 specimen each
qícǎo	

Preparation

(1) Pulverize the nine ingredients above and combine with honey [to form pills].

(2) A dose is seven pills the size of *wútóng* seeds. Increase this dose very gradually, measuring it by when you notice an effect.

鱉頭丸

治小兒痞氣，脅下腹中有積聚堅痛方。

鱉頭	一枚
蛀蟲	各十八銖
蟅蟲	
桃仁	
甘皮	半兩

（一）上五味，末之，蜜丸。服如小豆二丸，日
　　　三。

（二）大便不利，加大黃十八銖，以知為度。

VII.2.j Biētóu Wán (Turtle Head Pill)

Indication

A formula for small children, to treat *pǐ* glomus qì and the presence of accumulations, gatherings, hardening, and pain below the rib-sides and in the abdomen.

Ingredients

biētóu	1 specimen
méngchóng	
zhèchóng	18 *zhū* each
táorén	
gānpí	0.5 *liǎng*

Preparation

(1) Pulverize the five ingredients above and [process into] honey pills. Take two pills the size of mung beans, three times a day.

(2) If defecation is inhibited, add 18 *zhū* of *dàhuáng*, measuring it by when you notice an effect.

治小兒羸瘦惙惙，宜常服，不妨乳方。

甘草	五兩

（一）末之，蜜丸。

（二）一歲兒如小豆十丸，日三。服盡即更合。

VII.2.k Unnamed Formula[13]

Indication

A formula for small children, to treat marked emaciation and tiredness. It is appropriate to give this formula constantly and to not restrict breastfeeding.[14]

Ingredients

gāncǎo	5 liǎng

Preparation

(1) Pulverize it and [process it into] honey pills.

(2) For a child of one *suì*, give ten pills the size of mung beans, three times a day. When you have used up all the doses, immediately compound another [batch].

---

13   At first glance, the location of this formula here in the chapter on "Aggregations, Binds, Distension, and Fullness" seems a bit startling, since it clearly does not address these conditions. Moreover, the formula is not included in the chapter with this title in the *Sūn Zhēn Rén* edition, which predates the involvement of Lín Yì and his team of editors in the Sòng dynasty. Following the line of reasoning suggested by the *Yǎn Yì* commentary below, the Sòng editors most likely placed the formula here not to address the main conditions addressed in this chapter but as a treatment to mitigate the negative iatrogenic effects of the harsh down-draining formulas that precede it here.

14   不妨乳 bù fáng rǔ: This phrase could also be read quite differently as "There is no harm in breastfeeding." My reading is based on the context of the phrase in this formula. While 妨 on its own means "obstacle" or "to interfere with," the combination 不妨 has the idiomatic meaning of "there is no harm in" or "you may as well…".

《衍義》

(一) 牛黃丸為高梁者設，芒硝紫丸為藜藿者
　　 設。

(二) 方中牛黃除熱痰，療驚癎；真珠定神志，
　　 安魂魄；杏仁搜痰飲，下逆氣；巴豆逐乳
　　 癖，盪冷積；附子破症堅，散積聚，總行
　　 辛溫之力，以行寒降之用也。

(三) 芒硝紫丸方中芒硝以代真珠之滌熱，大
　　 黃、甘遂以代牛黃之盪實，半夏以代附子
　　 之破結，在粗屬之子，原無藉於峻溫也。

Commentary VII.2k ◂ Julian Scott

"...distinguished taste buds of the wealthy". I love this description of a fuss-pot who has never been made to eat anything that is not fancy. Matters are very different for the families where there is not enough food. Besides the difficulty in getting the pampered children to take unpleasant medicine, there is the issue of the nature of the food accumulating in the abdomen. In the wealthy families this will be rich, refined food, while in the poor families this is food full of fiber.

Yǎn Yì (Expanded Meaning)

(1) Niúhuáng Wán   is designed for the distinguished taste buds of the wealthy while Mángxiāo Zǐ Wán is designed for paupers used to simple and coarse foods.[15]

(2) In the formula [for Niúhuáng Wán), *niúhuáng* eliminates heat phlegm and cures fright seizures. *Zhēnzhū* settles the spirit and will and quiets the hún and pò souls. *Xìngrén* tracks down phlegm rheum and moves counterflow qì down. *Bādòu* expels milk aggregations and flushes out accumulations of cold. *Fùzǐ* breaks up concretions and hardenings and dissipates accumulations and gatherings, summoning the force of its acrid warmth to carry out its effect of downbearing cold.

(3) In the formula for Mángxiāo Zǐ Wán, *mángxiāo* is used as a substitute for *zhēnzhū* to scrub away heat, *dàhuáng* and *gānsuì* are used as substitutes for *niúhuáng* to flush

---

15   Literally translated, the line reads: "Niúhuáng Wán   is designed for those who [eat] sorghum while Mángxiāo Zǐ Wán is designed for those who [eat] wild greens." My fanciful translation of 高粱 ("sorghum") and 藜藿 ("lamb's quarters and other wild greens") as "distinguished taste buds of the wealthy" and "paupers used to simple and coarse foods" is based on the historical precedent of using these terms to refer to the fancy and refined foods of the wealthy and the simple meager diet of those who are forced by poverty to scavenge in nature for wild (and free) foods, respectively. It is ironic that in our modern times the relationship between economic status and access to natural foods and fresh vegetables seems to be the exact opposite. Especially in the United States, convenient access to fresh and organically grown greens, whole grain products, and minimally processed foods is often restricted to those with the wallet to shop at trendy health food markets or the space and leisure time to grow and harvest their own vegetables. As such, we may want to rethink the patient population that these two formulas are indicated for.

（四）其治八歲已上十五歲已下兒熱結痰實，食
減自下，並用芍藥、梔子、知母、大黃、
柴胡、升麻、黃芩、竹葉，一派清熱之
藥，但熱甚則用黃連、枯梗、細辛，痰多
則用枳實、杏仁、生薑。

（五）原不必以歲數拘也。

（六）牛黃雙丸以有心腹陽分之痛，故於牛黃丸
中除去附子，參入紫丸中甘遂，佐芍藥、
黃芩以盪實熱之固結。

out repletion, and *bànxià* is used as a substitute for *fùzǐ* to break up binds. Given the presence of the crude and formidable seeds,[16] [the formula] originally does not [have to] rely on the fierce warmth [of fuzi?].[17]

(4) The two [unnamed] treatments for heat binds and phlegm repletion with reduced eating and spontaneous bowel movements in children between the ages of eight and fifteen *suì* both use *sháoyào, zhīzhǐ, zhīmǔ, dàhuáng, cháihú, shēngmá, huángqín,* and *zhúyè,* which are all in the category of heat-clearing medicinals. Nevertheless, if the heat is severe, use *huánglián, jiégěng,* and *xìxīn,* and if the phlegm is predominant, use *zhǐshí, xìngrén,* and *shēngjiāng.*

(5) Originally, it is not necessary to restrict [their clinical application] to this age group.

(6) Niúhuáng Shuāng Tāng takes the presence of pain in the yáng aspect of the heart and abdomen as the reason to remove *fùzǐ* from the formula for Niúhuáng Wán and [instead] add *gānsuì* from the formula for Mángxiāo Zǐ Wán, with the assistance of *sháoyào* and *huángqín,* to flush out the solid binds of repletion heat.

---

16 Presumably a reference to the ingredients *bādòu* and *xìngrén*, which are found in both formulas. Alternatively, this line could be read as "In coarse and stern children,…"

17 This is my best guess for this somewhat obscure line. Other versions of Niúhuáng Wán exist that do not contain *bādòu* and *xìngrén* but I have not been able to find any formulas specifically named Niúhuáng Wán that pre-date the *Qiān Jīn Fāng*. In volume 14 of the *Qiān Jīn Fāng*, a "Nine Ingredient Niúhuáng Wán" (九物牛黃丸) is indicated specifically for men for a condition described as "wanting to die when encountering demons and goblins and wanting to run away when seeing something frightful or terrifying" (得鬼魅欲死，所見惊怖欲走) and aiming at expelling evil and settling fright. This formula does not contain *bādòu* or *xìngrén*, but whether the present line is a reference to this formula is impossible to determine with certainty.

（七）牛黃鱉甲丸以有癖實壯熱，故於後鱉甲丸
中除去庶蟲、蟅蟲啖血之味，參入牛黃、
厚朴、麥曲、枳實、川芎等味，以滌除痰
癖。

（八）二方俱參入桂、姜，以鼓牛黃、大黃、鱉
甲、芍藥之力也。

（九）芫花丸中只用雄黃一味，不特振芫花、大
黃、黃芩下奪之威，其宿蘊之積，亦得從
之下達矣。

（十）真珠丸方即於牛黃丸中專取真珠、巴豆二
味，又於雙紫丸中擇取蕘仁以佐巴豆，門
冬以佐真珠，藥品越減而功用越專矣。

（十一）鱉頭丸專取啖血之品，以攻血為務，乃
抵當湯、下淤血湯之變方，非若鱉甲丸之
於攻積藥中，兼行破血也。

(7) Niúhuáng Biējiǎ Wán takes the presence of aggregations and repletion with vigorous heat [effusion] as the reason to modify the formula below for Biējiǎ Wán, eliminating the blood-consuming ingredients *zhèchóng* and *qícǎo* but adding the ingredients *niúhuáng, hòupò, màiqū, zhǐshí,* and *chuānxiōng,* to flush out the phlegm aggregations.

(8) Both formulas include *guìxīn* and *gānjiāng* to arouse the strength of *niúhuáng, dàhuáng, biējiǎ,* and *sháoyào.*

(9) In the formula for Yuánhuā Wán, the single ingredient *xiónghuáng* is used not only to arouse the down-forcing might of *yuánhuā, dàhuáng,* and *huángqín.* In addition, it successfully causes the abiding smoldering accumulations to be moved down and expelled along with them.

(10) The formula for Zhēnzhū Wán has specifically taken the two ingredients *zhēnzhū* and *bādòu* from the formula for Niúhuáng Wán, while also selecting *ruǐhérén* and *màiméndōng* from the formula for Shuāng Zǐ Wán to assist *bādòu* and *zhēnzhū* respectively. The fewer medicinal ingredients a formula contains, the more specific its applications are.

(11) Biētóu Wán specifically uses blood-consuming substances to carry out the task of attacking blood. It is in fact a modification of the formulas Dǐdàng Tāng and Xià Yūxuè Tāng. Unlike Biējiǎ Wán, which places the accumulation-attacking action at center stage, it combines all its forces to break blood.

（十二）一味甘草蜜丸治小兒贏瘦，必因巴豆、
　　　　甘遂、大黃、牛黃等傷犯胃氣，而致惵惵
　　　　不安，故不借它藥，但取解藥毒。

（十三）若非藥蠱，與方無預。

(12) The marked emaciation in small children that the single-ingredient *gāncǎo* honey pills treat must be a condition that is caused by ingredients like *bādòu*, *gānsuì*, *dàhuáng*, and *niúhuáng*, which have damaged stomach qì and caused tiredness and unease. [This formula] therefore does not rely on any other medicinals but only focuses on resolving the toxins of these medicinals.

(13) If [the condition] is not a case of medicinal or *gǔ* poisoning,[18] administering this formula will cause no satisfaction.

---

18 The term here used to connote poisoning, namely 蠱 *gǔ*, literally refers to a specific type of poisoning, performed intentionally by people with harmful intentions by combining a variety of insect poisons to create dreadful chronic conditions of often hidden causation, which are therefore notoriously difficult to treat. Here it is most likely used simply to emphasize the chronic and deep-lying nature of conditions that are caused by iatrogenesis. It is, however, possible that the formula can also be used to treat *gǔ* poisoning, but is not useful for any other sort of poisoning.

桂心橘皮湯

治小兒五六日不食，氣逆方。

桂心	半兩
橘皮	三兩
成簟薚	五兩
黍米	五合
人參	半兩

（一）上五味，咬咀，以水七升先煮藥，煎取二升。

（二）次下薚、米，米熟藥成，稍稍服之。

桂心橘皮湯《衍義》

（一）桂心、人參、黍米，俱溫理胃氣虛寒之藥。

（二）兼橘皮以發越參、米補益之性，更加成簟之薚專泄胸中逆上之滯氣也。

VII.3 Formulas for Inability to Eat Due to Qi Disharmony

VII.3.a Guìxīn Júpí Tāng (Cinnamon Bark and Tangerine Peel Decoction)

Indication

A formula for small children who have not eaten in five or six days and who are suffering from qì counterflow.

Ingredients

guìxīn	0.5 liǎng
júpí	3 liǎng
xièbái that has leafed out	5 liǎng
shǔmǐ	5 gě
rénshēn	0.5 liǎng

Preparation

(1) Pound the five ingredients above. First decoct the medicinal ingredients[19] in 7 shēng of water until reduced to 2 shēng.

(2) Next add the xièbái and shǔmǐ. When the shǔmǐ is cooked, the medicine is done. Give it [to the patient] little by little.

---

19 I.e, guìxīn, júpí, and rénshēn.

Guìxīn Júpí Tāng (Cinnamon Bark and Tangerine Peel Decoction) Yǎn Yì (Expanded Meaning)

(1) Guìxīn, rénshēn, and shǔmǐ are all medicinals for warming the interior and [treating] stomach qì vacuity cold.

(2) The combination with júpí brings out and develops the supplementing and boosting nature of rénshēn and shǔmǐ, and the addition of leafed-out xièbái specifically discharges stagnant qì that has ascended counterflow in the lung.

地黃丸

治少小胃氣不調，不嗜食，生肌肉方。

乾地黃	各一兩六銖
大黃	
茯苓	十八銖
當歸	各半兩
柴胡	
杏仁	

（一）上六味，末之，以蜜丸如麻子大。

（二）服五丸，日三服。

VII.3.b Dìhuáng Wán (Rehmannia Pill)

Indication

A formula for children, to treat lack of attunement in the qì of the stomach with lack of appetite, by engendering flesh.

Ingredients

gandìhuáng	1 *liǎng* 6 *zhū* each
dàhuáng	
fúlíng	18 *zhū*
dāngguī	0.5 *liǎng* each
cháihú	
xìngrén	

Preparation

(1) Pulverize the six ingredients above and [form into] honey pills the size of hemp seeds.

(2) Take five pills per dose, three doses a day.

地黃丸《衍義》

(一) 此專療胃中氣血不調，飲食不為肌肉，故
專取地黃湯，傷中逐血。

(二) 當歸治傷寒熱和脾，柴胡升少陽生氣，杏
仁下胸中逆氣，大黃滌六腑實熱，茯苓守
五臟真氣也。

Dìhuáng Wán (Rehmannia Pill) *Yǎn Yì* (Expanded Meaning)

(1) This treatment specifically cures disharmony of qì and blood in the stomach and failure of food and drink to generate flesh. Therefore it specifically chooses Dìhuáng Tāng for damage to the center and expelling blood.[20]

(2) *Dāngguī* treats damage from cold and heat and harmonizes the spleen; *cháihú* upbears Shàoyáng and engenders qì; *xìngrén* brings down counterflow qì in the chest; *dàhuáng* flushes out repletion heat from the six bowels; and *fúlíng* safeguards the true qì of the five viscera.

---

20   逐血 *Zhú xuè* here refers to the intentional elimination of pathogenic blood, such as after childbirth in the formula for Zhú Xuè Tiáo Zhōng Dìhuáng Jiǔ 逐血調中地黃酒 (Blood-Expelling Center-Harmonizing Rehmannia Liquor).

馬通粟丸

治少小脅下有氣，內痛，喘逆，氣息難，往來寒熱，贏瘦不食方。

馬通中粟	十八銖
杏仁	各半兩
紫菀	
細辛	
石膏	各六銖
秦艽	
半夏	
茯苓	
五味子	

（一）上九味，末之，蜜丸。

（二）服如小豆十丸，日三服，不知加至二十丸。

VII.3.c Mătōngsù Wán (Horse Manure Grain Pill)

Indication

A formula for children, to treat presence of qì below the ribsides with internal pain, panting and counterflow, difficulty breathing, intermittent [aversion to] cold and heat [effusion], marked emaciation, and not eating.

Ingredients

mătōngzhōngsù (grain found in horse manure)	18 *zhū*
xìngrén	0.5 *liăng* each
zĭwăn	
xìxīn	
shígāo	6 *zhū* each
qínjiāo	
bànxià	
fúlíng	
wŭwèizĭ	

Preparation

(1) Pulverize the nine ingredients above and [form into] honey pills.

(2) Take ten pills about the size of mung beans per dose, three doses per day. If you do not notice [any effect], increase the dosage to a maximum of twenty pills.

馬通粟丸《衍義》

（一）馬通止血解毒，而馬通中粟專散胃中積
　　　垢。

（二）杏仁、細辛、紫菀祛風利氣，茯苓、半夏
　　　利水豁痰，石膏、五味化熱收津。

（三）聚散氣調，痰清熱化，而津自回矣。

Mǎtōng Sù Wán (Horse Manure Grain Pill) *Yǎn Yì* (Expanded Meaning)

(1) Horse manure stanches bleeding and resolves toxin, and the grains found in horse manure specifically dissipate accumulated filth in the stomach.

(2) *Xìngrén, xìxīn,* and *zǐwǎn* dispel wind and disinhibit qì. *Fúlíng* and *bànxià* disinhibit water and sweep away phlegm. *Shígāo* and *wǔwèizǐ* transform heat and astringe the liquids.

(3) When gatherings are dissipated, qì is attuned, phlegm is cleared, and heat is transformed, the liquids turn back around on their own.

治小兒下痢，腹大且堅方。

以故衣帶多垢者切一升，水三升，煮取一升，分三服。

腹上摩衣中白魚，亦治陰腫。

治少小腹脹滿方。

燒父母指甲灰，乳頭上飲之。

Commentary VII.4.a,e ᴥ Julian Scott

Fullness and distension can arise when the intestinal flora are out of balance. The prescriptions, though not in accord with modern ideas of hygiene, would certainly have the effect of introducing new bacteria. In the West we call these medicines 'probiotics'.

VII.4 Formulas for Abdominal Distention

VII.4.a

Indication

A formula for small children to treat diarrhea and dysentery[21] and an abdomen that is both enlarged and hard.

Preparation

Take an old cloth belt that has a lot of filth on it and cut up one *shēng*. Decoct in three *shēng* of water until reduced to 1 *shēng*. Divide into three doses.

VII.4.b Another formula:

Massage the top of the abdomen with silverfish.[22] This also treats swelling of the genitals.

VII.4.c

Indication

A formula for children, to treat abdominal Distension and fullness.

Preparation

Char fingernails from the [child's] mother and father into ashes, apply to the nipple of the [mother's or wetnurse's] breast, and have [the child] drink [and thereby ingest] it.

---

21   While some editions have 不痢 *bú lì* ("no dysentery") here instead, I follow the more logical reading. Unfortunately, this formula is not found in the *Sūn Zhēn Rén* edition, so we cannot use that text for confirmation.

22   See note on "white fish inside clothing" in *Venerating the Root, Part One* p. 249.

韭根汁和豬脂煎，細細服之。

車轂中脂和輪下土如彈丸，吞之立愈。

米粉、鹽等分，炒變色，腹上摩之。

《衍義》

（一）取爪甲肝氣之餘，以疏脾土之滯。

（二）韭根和豬脂以通腸胃之結。

（三）車脂和輪下土以疏土氣之壅。

（四）米鹽炒摩腹上，以調水土之通。

VII.4.d Another formula:

Combine chive root juice with pig lard and simmer it. Give this [to the patient] in very small amounts.

VII.4.e Another formula:

Mix grease from the center of the hub of a cart wheel with dirt from below the wheel and make pellet-sized pills. Swallowing these will cause immediate recovery.

VII.4.f Another formula:

Take equal amounts of rice flour and salt and toast until [the mixture] changes color. Massage [the child with] this on top of the abdomen.

Yǎn Yì (Expanded Meaning)

(1) Being the surplus of liver qì, fingernails are used to course the stagnation of spleen earth.

(2) The combination of chive root and pig lard is used to open up binds in the intestines and stomach.

(3) Cart grease mixed with dirt from underneath the tires is used to course the congestion of earth qì.

(4) Massaging the child's abdomen with toasted rice and salt attunes the free flow of water and earth.

當歸丸

（一）治小兒胎寒，口啼，腹中痛，舌上黑青，
　　　涎下方。

（二）一名黑丸。

Commentary VII.5.a ❧ **Julian Scott**

A common cause of fetal cold in our society is the excessive consumption of cold foods such as yoghurt and bananas during pregnancy. Another cause may be the use of anesthetics in childbirth and of antibiotics in general.

VII.5 Formulas for Fetal Cold and Abdominal Pain

VII.5.a Dāngguī Wán (Chinese Angelica Pill)

Indication

(1) A formula for small children, to treat fetal cold with a hunched-over posture and crying,[23] abdominal pain, black or blue-green [color] on the top of the tongue, and drooling.[24]

(2) Another name [for this formula] is Black Pill.[25]

---

23 The *Zhū Bìng Yuán Hòu Lùn* explains the symptom of 口啼 as follows: "If the mother during pregnancy has suffered damage from wind cold and evil qì entered the womb, this has damaged the child's viscera and bowels. After birth, the evil that is inside the child's abdomen stirs and struggles with right qì, causing abdominal pain. This causes the child to bend over and arch backwards, pant, and cry." See *Zhū Bìng Yuán Hòu Lùn*, vol. 47, entry on "(口匽) 啼." The entry following this one explains fetal cold (胎寒 *tāi hán*) as follows: "If the mother has contracted an excessive amount of cold while the baby is still in the womb, and the cold qì has entered the womb, this damages the child's intestines and stomach. Therefore, after the child is born, cold qì only sits in the region of the child's intestines and stomach. The symptoms of this condition are coldness in the child's intestines and abdomen, inability to transform breast milk or food, possibly abdominal Distension, or occasional grain diarrhea, causing the child's facial complexion to turn greenish white, and occasional crying."

24 In all modern editions, the last two phrases are punctuated differently as 舌上黑，青涎下方. This would translate as "blackness on top of the tongue and drooling of green-blue saliva." My reasons for disagreeing with the modern editors here is that 1) it makes more clinical sense to have a green-blue tongue than green-blue saliva, and 2) the rhythm of the language.

25 In some editions, including the *Sūn Zhēn Rén* edition, this second line is identified as an editorial comment, so it was most likely added by the editorial team around Lín Yì during the Sòng dynasty.

當歸	九銖
吳茱萸*	各半兩
蜀椒	
細辛	各十八銖
乾薑	
附子	
狼毒	九銖
豉	七合
巴豆	十枚

（一）上九味，搗七種下篩，秤藥末令足，研巴
豆如膏，稍稍納末，搗令相得。

（二）蜜和，桑杯盛，蒸五升米飯下，出搗一千
杵。

（三）一月兒服如黍米一丸，日一夜二，不知稍
加，以知為度。

（四）亦治水癖。

Ingredients

dāngguī	9 *zhū*
*wúzhūyú**	0.5 *liǎng* each
shǔjiāo	
xìxīn	18 *zhū* each
gānjiāng	
fùzǐ	
lángdú	9 *zhū*
chǐ	7 *gě*
bādòu	10 pieces

*Editorial note: Another version has *xìngrén* instead.

Preparation

(1) Of the nine ingredients above, pound the first seven and sift them. Measure the powdered medicinals on a scale and make sure you have sufficient amounts. Grind the *bādòu* into a paste-like consistency and little by little add it to the powder. Pound it again until it is thoroughly combined.

(2) Mix with honey and fill in a mulberry-wood cup.[26] Steam it under 5 *shēng* of rice until the rice is cooked. Take it out and pound it with a pestle a thousand times.

(3) For a child of one month, a dose is one pill the size of a millet grain. Give one pill during the day and two at night. If you don't notice [an effect], increase the dosage gradually, measuring it by when you notice an effect.

(4) [This formula] also treats water aggregations.

---

26   I.e. a cup made of wood from mulberry trees.

馬齒礬丸

治小兒胎寒，口啼，驚癇腹脹，不嗜食，大便青黃，並大人虛冷內冷，或有實不可吐下方。

馬齒礬	一斤

（一）燒半日，以棗膏和。

（二）大人服如梧子二丸，日三；小兒以意減之。

（三）以腹內溫為度，有實實去，神妙。

馬齒礬丸《衍義》

皂礬煅赤，最散氣血結滯，今名棗礬丸是也。

VII.5.b Mǎchǐfán Wán (Unprocessed Alum Pills)

Indication

A formula for small children, to treat fetal cold with a hunched-over posture and crying, fright seizures, abdominal Distension, no desire for food, and green-blue or yellow feces. It is also indicated for adults as a treatment for vacuity cold and internal cold, possibly with the presence of repletion that cannot be [expelled by] vomiting or bowel movements.

Ingredients[27]

mǎchǐfán	1 *jīn*

Preparation

(1) Roast it for half a day and then combine it with jujube paste.

(2) For adults, give two pills the size of *wútóng* seeds, 3 times a day. For small children, reduce the dosage at your discretion.

(3) Use warmth inside the abdomen as your measure [that the medicine is working]. If there was repletion, this repletion will now be gone. Divinely subtle!

---

27 Under the entry for *báifán* (alum), Táo Hóngjǐng mentions in his *Běncǎo Jīng Jízhù* that the unprocessed version of *báifán* is called *mǎchǐfán*. Wiseman translates the more common term 皂礬 *zàofán* as "melanterite."

Mǎchǐfán Wán (Unprocessed Alum Pills) *Yǎn Yì* (Expanded Meaning)

Zàofán that is calcined until red is most effective at dissipating binds and stagnations of qì and blood. The modern formula called Zàofán Wán is identical with this formula here.

梨葉濃汁

治小兒忽患腹痛，天矯汗出，名曰胎寒方。

煮梨葉濃汁七合，可三四度飲之。

梨葉濃汁《衍義》

（一）梨性寒滑，而煨熟食之，則不傷脾胃。

（二）梨葉煮濃汁，可治小兒胎寒腹痛，當是棠
　　　梨之葉，以裳梨能溫胃也。

VII.5.c Líyè Nóng Zhī (Concentrated Pear Leaf Juice)

Indication

A formula for small children to treat sudden attacks of abdominal pain with twisting and sweating. The name [for this disease] is "fetal cold."

Preparation

Decoct pear leaves to produce 7 *gě* of a concentrated liquid. You can [make the patient] drink this in three or four portions.

Líyè Nóng Zhī (Concentrated Pear Leaf Juice) *Yǎn Yì* (Expanded Meaning)

(1) Pear is by its nature cold and slippery. And yet, if it is consumed after being baked and cooked, it does not harm the spleen and stomach.

(2) Pear leaves that are decocted into a concentrated liquid can treat fetal cold with abdominal pain in small children. You should use the leaves of *tánglí* (i.e., sweet crabapple). The reason for this is that *tánglí* is able to warm the stomach.

半夏丸

治小兒暴腹滿欲死方。

（一）半夏隨多少，微火炮之，搗末。

（二）酒和服如粟米粒大五丸，日三，立愈。

半夏丸《衍義》

半夏一味，專滌頑痰，火炮酒服治腹痛，全在炮治得宜。

VII.5.d Bànxià Wán (Pinellia Pill)

Indication

A formula for small children to treat fulminant abdominal fullness that is bringing the patient close to death.

Preparation

(1) Take an appropriate amount of *bànxià* and roast it over a small flame. Pound into a powder.

(2) Mix with liquor and take five pills about the size of millet grains per dose, three times a day. Immediate recovery will ensue.

Bànxià Wán (Pinellia Pill) *Yǎn Yì* **(Expanded Meaning)**

As a single ingredient, *bànxià* specifically flushes out obstinate phlegm. Its effect of treating abdominal pain when it is roasted over a fire and taken with liquor is entirely due to the fact that roasting has made it suitable as a treatment.

治小兒霍亂吐痢方。

人參	一兩
厚朴	各半兩
甘草	
白朮	十八銖

（一）上四味，㕮咀，以水二升二合，煮取半
　　　升。

（二）六十日兒服一合，百日兒分三服，期歲分
　　　二服。

（三）中間隔乳服之。

（四）乳母忌生冷、油膩等。

VII.6 Formulas for Cholera

VII.6.a Unnamed Formula

Indication

A formula for small children to treat cholera[28] with vomiting and dysentery.

Ingredients

rénshēn	1 liǎng
hòupò	0.5 liǎng each
gāncǎo	
báizhú	18 zhū

Preparation

(1) Pound the four ingredients above and decoct in 2 shēng and 2 gě of water until reduced to 0.5 shēng.

(2) For a child sixty days old, give 1 gě per dose; for a child a hundred days old, divide [the formula] into three doses. For a child older than a complete year, divide it into two doses.

(3) Have the child breastfeed in between doses.

(4) The wet nurse or nursing mother must avoid foods that are raw and cold, oily and rich, etc.[29]

---

28 I follow Nigel Wiseman in translating 霍亂 (literally, "sudden chaos") as "cholera" not because I agree with the modern biomedical and TCM definition of "cholera" or 霍亂 as an acute bacterial infection with *Vibrio cholerae*, but because the English term "cholera," like the historical Chinese meaning of 霍亂, also has a larger meaning of "any of several diseases of humans and domestic animals usually marked by severe gastrointestinal symptoms" (Merriam-Webster Collegiate Dictionary).

29 Editorial note: Other versions of the formula add 1 fēn of *gānjiāng* or 3 *fēn* of *shēngjiāng*.

藿香湯

治毒氣吐下，腹脹，逆害乳哺方。

藿香	一兩
生薑	三兩
青竹茹	各半兩
甘草	

（一）上四味，咬咀，以水二升，煮取八合。

（二）每服一合，日三。

（三）有熱加升麻半兩。

VII.6.b Huòxiāng Tāng (Agastache Decoction)

Indication

A formula to treat toxic qì with vomiting and diarrhea, abdominal Distension, and counterflow, harming [the infant's ability to] nurse or feed.

Ingredients

huòxiāng	1 *liǎng*
shēngjiāng	3 *liǎng*
qīngzhúrú	0.5 *liǎng* each
gāncǎo	

Preparation

(1) Pound the four ingredients above and decoct in 2 *shēng* of water until reduced to 8 *gě*.

(2) Take 1 *gě* per dose, three times a day.

(3) When heat is present, add 0.5 *liǎng* of *shēngmá*.

治孩子霍亂，已用立驗方。

人參	各半兩
蘆蘀	
扁豆藤	二兩
倉米	一撮

上四味，咬咀，以水二升，煮取八合，分溫服。

又方

人參	一兩
木瓜	一枚
倉米	一撮

上三味，咬咀，以水煮，分服，以意量之，立效。

VII.6.c Unnamed Formula

Indication

A formula to treat cholera in children, immediately effective as soon as it is used.

Ingredients

rénshēn	0.5 *liǎng* each
lútuò*	
biǎndòuténg	2 *liǎng*
cāngmǐ	1 *cuō*

Translator's note: More commonly called 蘆筍 *lúsǔn*, the edible young sprouts of reed.

Preparation

Pound the four ingredients above and decoct in 2 *shēng* of water until reduced to 8 *gě*. Divide [into portions] and take warm.

VII.6.dAnother formula

Ingredients

rénshēn	1 *liǎng*
mùguā	1 piece
cāngmǐ	1 *cuō*

Preparation

Pound the three ingredients above and decoct in water. Divide and take, measuring it at your discretion. Immediately effective!

治小兒霍亂方。

研尿滓，乳上服之。

又方
牛涎灌口中一合。

治少小吐痢方。

亂髮	半兩，燒
鹿角	六銖

上二味，末之，米汁服一刀圭，日三服。

VII.6.e Unnamed Formula

Indication
A formula to treat cholera in small children.

Preparation
Grind urinary calculi and have the child ingest them by applying them on the [mother's] breast.

VII.6.f Another formula

Pour 1 *gě* of ox saliva into [the child's] mouth.

VII.6.g

Indication
A formula to treat vomiting and dysentery in children.

Ingredients

luànfà	charred, 0.5 *liǎng*
lùjiǎo	6 *zhū*

Preparation
Pulverize the two ingredients above and take 1 *dāoguī* in rice liquid, three doses per day.

《衍義》

（一） 此於理中湯中，去乾薑之守中，易厚朴以洩滿，即四君子中去茯苓之淡滲，易厚朴以溫散。

（二） 藿香湯則專取竹茹之清胃，得藿香以正氣，甘草以和中，借生薑之辛散以定霍亂。

（三） 其人參、蘆蕚、藊豆藤、陳倉米專治霍亂止後，胃氣虛乏。

（四） 人參、木瓜、倉米專治霍亂轉筋，木瓜能於土中瀉木。

（五） 牛涎以滋坤土，涎乃脾津。

（六） 亂髮灰治五癃關格利小便。

（七） 鹿角走肝腎督脈，而有止漏下散惡血之功，血散漏止而吐痢瘥矣。

Yǎn Yì (Expanded Meaning)
[Commentary on Cholera Treatments]

(1) The formula [for cholera listed under VII.6.a above] has removed the center-guarding action of *gānjiāng* from Lǐzhōng Tāng and substituted *hòupò* in order to drain fullness. It is also [related to] Sìjūnzǐ Tāng, having removed the bland percolating action of *fúlíng* and substituted *hòupò* to warm and dissipate.

(2) Huòxiāng Tāng specifically chooses *zhúrú* for its stomach-clearing effect and obtains *huòxiāng* to make qì right and *gāncǎo* to harmonize the center. It takes advantage of the acrid dissipating nature of *shēngjiāng* to settle the cholera.

(3) The [next formula's ingredients] *rénshēn, lútuó, biǎndòuténg,* and *chéncāngmǐ* specifically treat the state after cholera has stopped, when stomach qì is deficient and exhausted.

(4) *Rénshēn, mùguā,* and *cāngmǐ* specifically treat the cramping of sinews in cholera, with *mùguā* being able to drain wood from within earth.

(5) Ox saliva is used to enrich *kūn* earth, with saliva being the liquid associated with the spleen.

(6) *Luànfà* ash treats the five types of dribbling urinary block and block and repulsion, by disinhibiting urine.

(7) *Lùjiǎo* runs into the liver, kidney, and Dūmài channels and also has the merit of checking leaking below and dissipating malign blood. Once the blood is dissipated and the leaking checked, the vomiting and dysentery are cured!

又方：熱牛屎含之。

又方：燒特豬屎，水解取汁，少少服之。

治小兒癖，灸兩乳下一寸各三壯。

Commentary VII.6 Another Formula ◄ Julian Scott

Regarding the advice to feed the child ox or pig excrement, see my note above on probiotics (on the formulas for VII.4.a and e, p. 202). There is an interesting parallel with the animal world in that the mother elephant feeds her calf excrement to give the calf the bacteria necessary to digest her rather rough diet.

Another formula: Heat cow manure and have [the child] hold it in the mouth.[30]

Another formula: Char manure from a female pig, dissolve it in water, and take the liquid. Make the patient ingest it little by little.

VII.7 MOXIBUSTION

To treat aggregations in small children, burn three cones of moxa 1 *cùn* below the breasts on both sides.

---

30   Editorial Note: "Another formula calls for *niúxī* instead." The reason for this textual divergence is the fact that in Chinese, the compound terms for "cow manure" (牛屎 *niúshǐ*) and the medicinal *niúxī* (牛膝 *niúxī*, lit. "cow's knee") are quite similar, especially in sound.

CHAPTER EIGHT: WELLING ABSCESSES, FLAT ABSCESSES, AND SCROFULA

癰疽瘰癧第八

(1 essay, 73 formulas, 1 moxibustion method)

漏蘆湯

治小兒熱毒癰疽，赤白諸丹毒，瘡癤方。

VIII.1 Lòulú Tāng (Rhaponticum Decoction)

Indication

A formula for small children, to treat heat toxin flat- and well-ing-abscesses, the various kinds of red and white cinnabar toxin,[1] and sores and boils.

---

1 It is important to recognize here again that the term cinnabar (丹 *dān*) in the present context does not refer literally to the effects of consumption of mercuric sulfide but to a pediatric condition that has nothing to do with the physical substance cinnabar. While even some pediatric formulas in classical Chinese medicine do include cinnabar as a medicinal ingredient, research has shown that the form of mercury that is used therapeutically in Chinese medicine (mercuric sulfide, which is insoluble and has a very low bioavailability when not heated) does not share the highly toxic properties of some of its mercuric relatives, such as methyl mercury or mercury vapor. Inorganic mercury salts "collect in the kidney and are excreted in the urine and feces, with a half-life of about 2 months." See Liu, Shi, Yu, Goyer, and Waalkes, "Mercury in traditional medicines: Is cinnabar toxicologically similar to common mercurials?" *Exp. Biol. Med* (Maywood), July 2008; 233(7): 810–817. Actual poisoning from cinnabar is therefore possible, but only in the context of vastly excessive consumption or during processing such as heating. For more information on *dān* as a pediatric disease, see *Venerating the Root, Part One*, p. 27, note 3. According to the *Zhū Bìng Yuán Hòu Lùn*, vol. 31, *dān* is a condition that causes the body to suddenly turn red, "as if painted with cinnabar," arising in the hands and feet or on the abdomen, and always caused by wind heat toxin. If not treated immediately, it will develop into unbearable pain and will eventually fester and release large amounts of blood and pus. The *Zhū Bìng Yuán Hòu Lùn* further warns that the condition is deadly once the toxin enters the abdomen, and is particularly dangerous in small children. Based on my cursory research, it seems unlikely that the condition can be equated with smallpox, as suggested by some authors, because smallpox did not become endemic in China until several centuries later. How the classical Chinese condition of *dān* relates to such biomedical conditions as erysipelas is beyond the framework of this book.

漏蘆	各六銖
連翹	
白薟	
芒硝	
甘草	
大黃	一兩
升麻	各九銖
枳實	
麻黃	
黃芩	

（一）上十味，咬咀，以水一升半煎取五合。

（二）兒生一日至七日，取一合分三服。八日至
十五日，取一合半分三服。十六日至二十
日，取二合分三服。二十日至三十日，取
三合分三服。三十日至　四十日，取五合分
三服。

（三）其丹毒須針鑱去血。

Ingredients

lòulú	
liánqiáo	
báiliǎn	6 *zhū* each
mángcǎo	
gāncǎo	
dàhuáng	1 *liǎng*
shēngmá	
zhǐshí	9 *zhū* each
máhuáng	
huángqín,	

Editorial comment: The *Zhǒu Hòu* uses *báiwēi* instead of *liánqiáo* and *sháoyào* in place of *mángxiāo*.

Preparation

(1) Pound the ten ingredients above and decoct in 1.5 *shēng* of water until reduced to 5 *gě*.

(2) For a child of one to seven days, give 1 *gě*, divided into three doses. For a child of eight to fifteen days, give 1.5 *gě*, divided into three doses. For a child of sixteen to twenty days, give 2 *gě*, divided into three doses. For a child of twenty to thirty days, give 3 *gě*, divided into three doses. For a child of thirty to fourty days, give 5 *gě*, divided into three doses.[2]

(3) For the cinnabar toxin, you must needle with a chisel needle to get rid of the blood.[3]

---

2 In the *Zhǒu Hòu Bèi Jí Fāng* 肘後備急方, [this formula] is for adults, using 2 *liǎng* of each [of the other] ingredients and 3 *liǎng* of *dàhuáng*, decocted in 1 *dǒu* of water until reduced to 3 *shēng* and divided into three doses.

3 Editorial comment: The *Jīng Xīn Lù* 經心錄 "Record Passing Through the Heart" does not use *liánqiáo* but includes *zhīmǔ*, *sháoyào*, and *xījiǎo*, all in equal amounts.

漏蘆湯《衍義》

（一）方以漏蘆立名，專取利竅解毒，表裡兼
　　　該，以洩其邪。

（二）升麻、白蘞助麻黃以開鬼門。

（三）枳實、芒硝助大黃以潔淨府。

（四）連翹、黃芩、甘草，則漏蘆之佐使也。

Lòulú Tāng (Rhaponticum Decoction) *Yǎn Yì* (Expanded Meaning)

(1) The formula is named after *lòulú*, which is chosen specifically to disinhibit the orifices and resolve toxin. It involves both the interior and exterior concurrently, to drain away the patient's evil.

(2) *Shēngmá* and *báiliǎn* assist *máhuáng* in opening the sweat pores.[4]

(3) *Zhǐshí* and *mángxiāo* assist *dàhuáng* in cleansing the urinary bladder.[5]

(4) *Liánqiáo*, *huángqín*, and *gāncǎo* serve as assistants and envoys to *lòulú*.

---

4 鬼門 *guǐmén*: This term literally means "ghost gates," but in medical contexts has the technical meaning of sweat pores. As such, the text here simply means that *shēngmá* and *báiliǎn* support the sweat-promoting effect of *máhuáng*. We know that 鬼門 was already used to refer to "sweat pores" in early medieval medical literature because of Wáng Bīng's 王冰 commentary on the following passage from the *Sù Wèn* 《素問：湯液醪醴論》："開鬼門，潔淨腑。" Wáng Bīng's commentary from 762 CE explains this line: "'Open the Ghost Gates' means 'open up the sweat pores to get rid of qì. 'Cleanse the Pure Palace' refers to draining water from the urinary bladder' (開鬼門，是啟玄府遣氣也；潔淨腑，謂瀉膀胱水去也。).

5 淨腑 *jìngfǔ* : This term means literally "clean bowel," but refers also specifically to the urinary bladder in medical contexts.

五香連翹湯

治小兒風熱毒腫，腫色白，或有惡核瘰癧，附骨癰疽，節解不舉，白丹走竟身中，白疹瘙不已方。

Commentary VIII.2 ◆ Sabine Wilms

瘰癧 *luǒlì*: With some hesitation, I follow Wiseman's Practical Dictionary in translating this term as "scrofula." One could make a case for translating it simply as "swollen lymph nodes," but that does not seem quite specific enough. While the English term is used most often to refer to swellings that are due to infection with mycobacterium tuberculosis, scrofula can be caused by any infection from mycobacteria. The word scrofula is derived from the diminutive of the Latin scrofa, meaning sow. The earliest received reference to the Chinese term 瘰癧 is found in the *Líng Shū*: "The Yellow Emperor asked Qí Bó: 'Regarding the presence of cold and heat *luǒlì* at the neck or in the armpits, what kind of qì causes their formation?' Qí Bó answered: 'This is always the toxic qì of mouse fistula cold or heat, which lodges in the vessels and does not leave." 黃帝問于歧伯曰：寒熱瘰癧在於頸腋者，皆何氣使生？歧伯曰：此皆鼠瘻寒熱之毒氣也，留於脈而不去者也。The *Shuō Wén* in turn defines 瘻 as "swellings on the neck." According to the *Nèi Jīng Cí Diǎn* 內經辭典 (Dictionary of the Inner Classic), 瘰癧 refers to large and small nodes between the size of jujube pits and plums that are connected to each other and form in the area of the neck and below the armpit. When they eventually erupt, they are called "mouse fistula."

VIII.2 Wǔ Xiāng Liánqiáo Tāng (Five Fragrances Forsythia Decoction)

Indication

A formula for small children, to treat wind heat toxin swelling, [manifesting with] swelling and a white complexion,[6] or possibly with malign nodes and scrofula, flat- and welling-abscesses attached to the bones, separated joints preventing the patient from lifting [the limbs], white cinnabar[7] running all throughout the body, and white papules that itch incessantly.

---

6 I translate 腫色白 as "swelling with a white complexion" instead of as "white-colored swelling" based on the following description of the condition White Cinnabar (白丹 bái dān) in the *Zhū Bìng Yuán Hòu Lùn*: 疹 (sic. 疹) 起不痛不赤面白色 "papules rising that are neither painful nor red, and a white complexion in the face." See note 8 below.

7 白丹 bái dān: Literally translated, white cinnabar. This refers to a variety of neonatal dān (also known as "fetal toxin" 胎毒 tāi dú) that is characterized by a white facial complexion and associated with wind cold. The entry specifically on White *Dān* in the *Zhū Bìng Yuán Hòu Lùn* explains that this variety "first manifests with itching and pain, mild vacuity swelling that appears 'as if being blown [about by wind]', papules rising that are neither painful nor red, and a white complexion in the face. Because [the condition] is linked to wind cold, it turns the complexion white."

Commentary VIII.2 ⸱⸱ Julian Scott

Because of the association of the term "scrofula" with TB of the lymph glands in biomedicine, the translation of *luǒlì* as such is questionable. I don't know what the two characters meant in those days, but in modern TCM, the term has a somewhat wider meaning than TB of the lymph glands, and includes just simple swelling of the lymph nodes, with or without discharge. It may be caused by a lingering pathogenic factor, or even stagnation of qi. For example, I knew a person (fortunately not a patient) who was so angry at one time in his life that the glands in his groin (on the Liver channel) swelled up enormously and discharged pus.

青木香	
熏陸香	
雞舌香	各六銖
沉香	
麻黃	
黃芩	
大黃	二兩
麝香	三銖
連翹	
海藻	
射乾	各半兩
升麻	
枳實	
竹瀝	三合

（一）上十四味，咬咀，以水四升，煮藥減半，
納竹瀝，煮取一升二合。

（二）兒生百日至二百日，一服三合。二百日至
期歲，一服五合。

Ingredients

qīngmùxiāng	
xūnlùxiāng	
jīshéxiāng	6 *zhū* each
chénxiāng	
*máhuáng**	
huángqín	
dàhuáng	2 *liǎng*
shèxiāng	3 *zhū*
liánqiáo	
hǎizǎo	
shègān	0.5 *liǎng* each
shēngmá	
zhǐshí	
zhúlì	3 *gě*

*Editorial comment: Another [version of this] formula does not use *máhuáng*.

Preparation

(1) Of the fourteen ingredients above, pound the medicinals and decoct them in 4 *shēng* of water until reduced to half. Add the *zhúlì* and decoct [again] until reduced to 1 *shēng* and 2 *gě*.

(2) For children one hundred to two hundred days old, one dose is 3 *gě*. For children two hundred days to a full year old, one dose is 5 *gě*.

五香連翹湯 《衍義》

（一）風熱毒腫色白，明是氣滯痰結，故需五香
達竅為主。

（二）其麻黃佐升麻以開肌膚，枳實佐大黃以盪
腸胃，黃芩佐連翹以散風熱，海藻佐射乾
以軟堅結，竹瀝專行經絡，以開痰氣也。

Wǔ Xiāng Liánqiáo Tāng (Five Fragrances Forsythia Decoction) *Yǎn Yì* (Expanded Meaning)

(1) Wind heat toxic swelling with a white complexion is obviously a sign of qì stagnation and phlegm binding. Therefore we need the five fragrances to outthrust the orifices as the rulers [in this formula].

(2) The *máhuáng* in this formula assists *shēngmá* in opening up the flesh and skin; *zhǐshí* assists *dàhuáng* in flushing out the intestines and stomach; *huángqín* assists *liánqiáo* in dissipating wind heat; and *hǎizǎo* assists *shègān* in softening hardenings and binds. *Zhúlì* specifically moves the channels and network vessels, to open up phlegm qì.

連翹丸

治小兒無故寒熱，強健如故，而身體頸項結核瘰癧，及心脅腹背裡有堅核不痛，名為結風氣腫方。

連翹	
桑白皮	
白頭翁	
牡丹	
防風	各一兩
黃柏	
桂心	
香豉	
獨活	
秦芃	
海藻	半兩

（一）上十一味，末之，蜜丸如小豆。

（二）三歲兒飲服五丸，加至十丸。五歲以上者，以意加之。

VIII.3 Liánqiáo Wán (Forsythia Pill)

Indication

A formula for small children, to treat cold and heat without any [apparent] cause, with strength and good health as before, but nodes and scrofula all over the body and on the nape and neck, as well as hard painless nodes inside the heart, rib-sides, abdomen, and back. This is called binding wind qì swelling.

Ingredients

liánqiáo	
sāngbáipí	
báitóuwēng	
mǔdān	
fángfēng	1 *liǎng* each
huángbò	
guìxīn	
xiāngchǐ	
dúhuó	
qínjiāo	
hǎizǎo	0.5 *liǎng*

Preparation

(1) Pulverize the eleven ingredients above and form honey pills about the size of mung beans.

(2) For a child of three *suì*, give five pills per dose in liquid, increasing the dosage to up to ten pills. For a child older than five *suì*, increase [the dosage] at your discretion.

連翹丸《衍義》

（一）方中防風、白頭翁、香豉以散風毒，連
　　　翹、秦艽、桑皮、海藻以散氣腫。

（二）然風藥、氣藥非得血藥，不能透達營分。

（三）以散結核又須黃柏、桂心寒熱交攻。

（四）用牡丹者專和黃柏、桂心之寒熱也。

Liánqiáo Wán (Forsythia Pill) *Yǎn Yì* (Expanded Meaning)

(1) In the present formula, *fángfēng*, *báitóuwēng*, and *xiāng-chǐ* are used to dissipate wind toxin, while *liánqiáo*, *qín-jiāo*, *sāngpí*, and *háizǎo* are used to dissipate qì swelling.

(2) Nevertheless, if the wind medicinals and qì medic-inals[8] do not receive [the supportive effect] of blood medicinals, they are unable to break through and out-thrust the *yíng* [construction] level.

(3) To dissipate binds and nodes, you moreover need the cold and heat of *huángbò* and *guìxīn* for a joint offense.

(4) *Mǔdān* is used here specifically to harmonize the cold and heat of *huángbò* and *guìxīn*.

---

8 風藥，氣藥 *fēng yào, qì yào*: This refers to the medicinals that address the wind- and qì-related issues in this particular condition.

治丹毒，大赤腫，身壯熱，百治不折方。

寒水石	十六銖
石膏	十三銖
藍青	十二銖
犀角	各八銖
柴胡	
杏仁	
知母	十銖
甘草	五銖
羚羊角	六銖
芍藥	七銖
栀子	十一銖
黃芩	七銖
竹瀝	一升
生葛汁	四合，澄清
蜜	二斤

VIII.4 Formulas to Treat Cinnabar Toxin

VIII.4.a Unnamed Formula to Treat Cinnabar Toxin with Large Red Swelling and Vigorous Generalized Heat

Indication

A formula to treat cinnabar toxin with large red swelling and vigorous generalized heat, which a hundred treatments have been unable to break.

Ingredients

hánshuǐshí	16 *zhū*
shígāo	13 *zhū*
*lánqīng**	12 *zhū*
xījiǎo	8 *zhū* each
cháihú	
xìngrén	
zhīmǔ	10 *zhū*
gāncǎo	5 *zhū*
língyángjiǎo	6 *zhū*
sháoyào	7 *zhū*
zhīzhǐ	11 *zhū*
huángqín	7 *zhū*
zhúlì	1 shēng
shēnggézhī (i.e. fresh *gégēn* juice)	4 *gě*, allowed to settle and clear
fēngmì	2 *jīn*

*Editorial comment: In winter, use the dried herb.

（一）上十五味，㕮咀，以水五升並竹瀝煮取三
　　　升三合，去滓，納杏仁脂、葛汁、蜜，微
　　　火煎取二升。

（二）一二歲兒服二合，大者量加之。

麻黃湯

治小兒丹腫，及風毒風疹方。

麻黃	一兩半
獨活	各一兩
射乾	
甘草	
桂心	
青木香	
石膏	
黃芩	

（一）上八味，㕮咀，以水四升，煮取一升。

（二）三歲兒分為四服，日再。

Preparation

(1) Of the fifteen ingredients above, pound [the dry ingredients] and decoct them in 5 *shēng* of water together with the *zhúlì* until reduced to 3 *shēng* and 3 *gě*. Discard the dregs and add the *xìngrén* paste, *gégēn* juice, and honey. Brew over a small flame until reduced to 2 *shēng*.

(2) For a child of one to two *suì*, give 2 *gě* per dose. For an older child, increase the amount.

VIII.4.b Máhuáng Tāng (Ephedra Decoction)

Indication

A formula for small children, to treat cinnabar swelling as well as wind toxin and wind papules.

Ingredients

máhuáng	1.5 *liǎng*
dúhuó	
shègān	
gāncǎo	
guìxīn	1 *liǎng* each
qīngmùxiāng	
shígāo	
huángqín	

Preparation

(1) Pound the eight ingredients above and decoct in 4 *shēng* of water until reduced to 1 *shēng*.

(2) For a child of three *suì*, divide into four doses, given in two doses per day.

治小兒惡毒丹及風疹，麻黃湯方。

麻黃	各一兩
升麻	
葛根	
射乾	各半兩
雞舌香	
甘草	
石膏	半合

（一）上七味，咬咀，以水三升，煮取一升。

（二）三歲兒分三服，日三。

VIII.4.c Another Formula for Máhuáng Tāng (Ephedra Decoction)

Indication

A formula for small children, to treat malign poisoning from cinnabar, as well as wind papules.

Ingredients

máhuáng	1 *liǎng* each
shēngmá	
gégēn	
shègān	0.5 *liǎng* each
jīshéxiāng	
gāncǎo	
shígāo	0.5 *gě*

Preparation

(1) Pound the seven ingredients above and decoct in 3 *shēng* of water until reduced to 1 *shēng*.

(2) For a child of three *suì*, divide into three doses, given three times a day.

搨湯

治小兒數十種丹方。

大黃	各一兩
甘草	
當歸	
芎藭	
白芷	
獨活	
黃芩	
芍藥	
升麻	
沉香	
青木香	
木蘭皮	
芒硝	三兩

上十三味，咬咀，以水一斗一升，煮取四升，去
滓，納芒硝，以綿搵湯中，適寒溫搨之，乾則易
之，取瘥止。

VIII.4.d Tà Tāng (Rubbing⁹ Decoction)

Indication

A formula for small children, to treat the dozens of varieties of cinnabar.

Ingredients

dàhuáng	
gāncǎo	
dāngguī	
xiōngqióng	
báizhǐ	
dúhuó	1 *liǎng* each
huángqín	
sháoyào	
shēngmá	
chénxiāng	
qīngmùxiāng	
mùlánpí	
mángxiāo	3 *liǎng*

Preparation

Of the thirteen ingredients above, pound [the herbs] and decoct in 1 *dǒu* and 1 *shēng* of water until reduced to 4 *shēng*. Remove the dregs and add the *mángxiāo*. Take silk floss and submerge it in the decoction. Rub [the patient] down with this at a comfortable temperature. When [the floss] dries, change it. Stop when you have achieved recovery.

---

9 搨 *tà*: This character refers literally to the action of rubbing a sheet of paper over ink-covered stone inscriptions to produce a copy of the calligraphy on the paper.

（一）治小兒溺灶丹，初從兩股及臍間起，走入
　　　陰頭，皆赤方。

（二）桑根皮切一斗，以水二斗，煮取一斗，以
　　　洗浴之。

（一）治小兒丹毒方。

（二）搗慎火草，絞取汁，塗之良。

VIII.4.e Unnamed Formula to Treat "Urine Stove Cinnabar"

Indication

A formula for small children, to treat "urine stove cinnabar,"[10] which initially starts from the thighs or the umbilical area, runs into the tip of the penis,[11] and is marked by redness in all cases.

Ingredients and Preparation

Chop 1 *dǒu* of *sānggénpí* and decoct in 2 *dǒu* of water until reduced to 1 *dǒu*. Use this to wash it.[12]

VIII.4.f Unnamed Formula to Treat Cinnabar Toxin.

Indication

A formula for small children, to treat cinnabar toxin.[13]

Ingredients and Preparation

Pound *shènhuǒcǎo*[14] and wring it out to obtain the juice. Spreading this on the patient is excellent.

---

10 According to the chapter on "Treatments of Fire Cinnabar Patterns" in the *Lú Xìn Jīng*, Qí Bó explains to the Yellow Emperor that the various types of "fire cinnabar" can be diagnosed on the basis of their origin, and that "urine stove cinnabar" is differentiated by the fact that it starts from the ankles, while "spirit stove cinnabar," to give just one other example, starts from the abdomen.

11 陰頭 *yīn tóu*: Literally the "head of the genitals," this is a technical term that refers to either the penis as a whole or the tip thereof. As such, this formula appears to be indicated only for male patients.

12 The Chinese particle 之 is a direct object that can refer to either a person or a thing and can be singular or plural. I have therefore translated it literally as "it," so that readers can make up their own minds as to whether these instructions call for washing only the penis or the entire area affected. We can even translate it as "him," and read it in the sense of washing the entire patient.

13 Editorial comment: Formulas for [treating] cinnabar toxin [in adults] are all found in volume 22 of the *Bèi Jí Qiān Jīn Yào Fāng*.

14 This is an alternate name for the herb that is more commonly known as 景天 *jǐngtiān*. This herb is identified as Alpine Stonecrop or *Sedi Aizoon Herba* by Wiseman and as *Sedum Erythrostictum Miq.* in the *Zhōng Yào Dà Cí Diǎn*.

（一）治小兒赤游腫，若遍身，入心腹即殺人
　　　方。
（二）搗伏龍肝，末之，以雞子白和敷，乾易
　　　之。

白豆末，水和敷之，勿令乾。

治小兒半身皆紅赤，漸漸長引者方。

牛膝
甘草

上二味，咬咀，合得五升，以水八升，煮三沸，
去滓，和伏龍肝末敷之。

VIII.4.g Unnamed Formula to Treat Red Roaming Swelling

Indication

A formula for small children, to treat red roaming swelling. If this covers the entire body and enters the heart and abdomen, it will immediately kill the person.

Ingredients and Preparation

Crush *fúlónggān* and pulverize it. Combine it with egg white and spread it on [the affected area]. When [the mixture] is dry, change it.

Another Formula

Pulverize white beans and combine with water. Spread this on [the patient] and do not allow it to dry out.

VIII.4.h Unnamed Formula to Treat Strong Redness All Over Half the Body that Gradually Grows and Spreads.

Indication

A formula for small children, to treat strong redness all over half the body that gradually grows and spreads.

Ingredients

niúxī
gāncǎo

Preparation

Pound [equal amounts of] the two ingredients above and combine [a large enough amount] that you get 5 *shēng*. Decoct in 8 *shēng* of water, bringing it to a boil three times. Remove the dregs and combine with pulverized *fúlónggān*. Spread it on [the affected area].

治小兒身赤腫起者方。

熬米粉令黑，以唾和敷之。

| 伏龍肝 |
| 亂髮灰 |

上二味，末之，以膏和敷之。

治小兒猝腹皮青黑方。

（一）以酒和胡粉敷上。
（二）若不急治，須臾便死。

VIII.4.i Unnamed Formula to Treat Generalized Redness, Swelling, and Elevation.

Indication

A formula for small children, to treat generalized redness, swelling, and elevation.

Ingredients and Preparation

Toast rice flour until it is black. Mix this with saliva and spread it on [the affected area].

Another Formula

Ingredients

fúlónggān
luànfà, ashed

Preparation

Pulverize the two ingredients above and mix with grease. Spread it on [the affected area].

VIII.4.j Unnamed Formula for Small Children, to Treat Conditions Where the Skin over the Abdomen Suddenly Turns Green-blue or Black.

Ingredients and Preparation

(1) Mix *húfěn* into liquor. Spread it on top [of the abdomen].

(2) If you do not treat this with urgency, [the patient] will invariably die instantly.

又，灸臍上下左右去臍半寸，並鳩尾骨下一寸，凡五處，各三壯。

《衍義》

（一）丹毒總屬火證，故用寒水石、石膏、犀角、羚羊、柴胡、芩、梔，一派解毒散血清肝之劑，專治從內炘發之毒。

（二）麻黃湯方用麻黃、桂心、射乾、獨活，皆主外內合邪之證，以分解蘊熱之勢。

（三）其石膏、黃芩、青木香、甘草，仍不出乎正治之法也。

（四）其又方，則全從事於外解。升、葛、射乾即前方射乾、獨活佐黃芩之意。

（五）雞舌香即前方桂心導伏熱之意。

（六）石膏、甘草則與上二方無異也。

Another [Method]:

Burn moxa above and below and to the right and left of the navel, half a *cùn* away from the navel, as well as 1 *cùn* below the xiphoid process, in a total of five locations, three cones each.

Yǎn Yì (Expanded Meaning)

(1) Cinnabar toxin is always associated with fire patterns. Therefore we use *hánshuǐshí, shígāo, xījiǎo, língyáng, cháihú, huángqín,* and *zhīzhǐ,* all of which are in the single category of toxin-resolving blood-dissipating liver-clearing preparations, to specifically treat the toxin that is flaring up from the inside.

(2) The formula for Máhuáng Tāng uses *máhuáng, guìxīn, shègān,* and *dúhuó,* which are all indicated for patterns of combined internal and external evils, thereby separately resolving the force of brewing heat.

(3) The ingredients *shígāo, huángqín, qīngmùxiāng,* and *gāncǎo* in this formula do not deviate from this direct treatment method.

(4) The next formula [for Máhuáng Tāng] then focuses completely on external resolution. *Shēngmá, gégēn,* and *shègān* [here] have the same intent as *shègān* and *dúhuó* in the previous formula, namely to assist *huángqín.*

(5) *Jīshéxiāng* has the same intent as *guìxīn* in the previous formula, namely to abduct the deep-lying heat.

(6) *Shígāo* and *gāncǎo* are [used] no differently than in the previous two formulas.

（七）搨湯清解表裡熱毒，藥皆純良無奇。

（八）木蘭皮近世罕用，考諸《本經》治大熱在皮膚中，去面熱赤皰酒皶等證，使熱從皮腠而散也。

（九）一味桑根皮煮湯浴之，專取其散風熱也。

（十）慎火草絞汁塗之，專取其解火毒也。

（十一）伏龍肝末、雞子白和傳，專取其散虛熱也。

（十二）白豆與赤豆之狀不異，但色白至氣分，而解皮膚熱毒。

（十三）牛膝、甘草皆生用，煎取濃汁和伏龍肝末傳之，功用與伏龍肝和雞子白傳之不殊。

(7) The rubbing decoction clears and resolves heat toxin in the exterior and interior. The medicinal ingredients are all straight-forward and there is nothing strange about them.

(8) *Mùlánpí* is rarely used in modern times,[15] but an investigation of the *Shénnóng Běncǎo Jīng* [shows] that it treats great heat inside the skin and gets rid of patterns like heat in the face, red pimples, and liquor blotches, by causing the heat to dissipate through the skin's interstices.

(9) Washing the patient with a decoction prepared from the single ingredient *sānggénpí* specifically takes advantage of [this medicinal's ability] to dissipate wind heat.

(10) Applying the juice from wrung-out *shènhuǒcǎo* specifically takes advantage of this medicinal's [ability] to resolve fire toxin.

(11) Mixing *fúlónggān* with egg white and spreading it on the body specifically takes advantage of these ingredients' [ability] to dissipate vacuity heat.

(12) White beans are no different in shape from red beans, but the white ones reach the qì level and resolve heat toxin in the skin.

(13) Boiling down the juice from raw *niúxī* and *gāncǎo* until it is concentrated, mixing this with pulverized *fúlónggān*, and spreading it on [the affected area] is no different in effect than the application of *fúlónggān* mixed with egg white.

---

15 Note that "modern times" refers not to contemporary clinical practice, nor to Sūn Sīmiǎo's times, but to the time of composition of the *Qiān Jīn Fāng Yǎn Yì*, or in other words to Chinese clinical practice in the late seventeenth century.

（十四）熬米粉以唾和傅取米能長肉，黑能解毒也，與前治小兒小腹腫滿，用米鹽炒摩同意，以鹽能軟堅，同源異派。

（十五）伏龍肝、亂髮灰傅，與前和雞子白傅少異，以亂髮灰能散滯血也。

（十六）小兒卒腹皮青黑，用酒和胡粉傅，專取鉛性鎮攝火毒也。

(14) Applying a mixture of toasted rice flour and saliva utilizes the ability of rice to grow flesh and, when blackened, to resolve toxin. It has the same intent as the treatment in the previous chapter for lesser abdominal swelling and fullness in small children, where a mixture of rice and salt is fried and used to massage the patient, using the ability of salt to soften hardness. This is [like two rivers that] share the same source but have split off into different branches.

(15) The external application of *fúlónggān* and *luànfà* ashes differs slightly from the application of [*fúlónggān*] in a mixture with egg white above, because *luànfà* ashes are able to dissipate stagnant blood.

(16) When small children suddenly have the skin on their abdomen turn green-blue or black, applying a mixture of liquor and *húfěn* specifically takes advantage of the nature of lead to repress and contain fire toxin.

五香枳實湯

治小兒著風熱，(疒音)瘤堅麻豆粒，瘡癢搔之皮剝汁出，或遍身頭面年年常發者方。

青木香	九銖
麝香	六銖
雞舌香	各半兩
熏陸香	
沉香	
升麻	各一兩
黃芩	
白斂	
麻黃	
防風	各半兩
秦艽	
枳實	一兩半
大黃	一兩十八銖
漏蘆	半兩

VIII.5 Formulas for Sores from Wind Heat, Damp Heat, and Burns

VIII.5.a Wǔ Xiāng Zhǐshí Tāng (Five Fragrances Unripe Bitter Orange Decoction)

Indication

A formula for small children, to treat wind heat affliction, with dormant papules that are hard and resemble leprosy, sores that itch and ooze liquid when scratched until the skin breaks, and possibly consistent outbreaks all over the body and on the head and face for year after year.

Ingredients

qīngmùxiāng	9 zhū
shèxiāng	6 zhū
jīshéxiāng	0.5 liǎng each
xūnlùxiāng	
chénxiāng	
shēngmá	1 liǎng each
huángqín	
báiliǎn	
máhuáng	
fángfēng	0.5 liǎng each
qínjiāo	
zhǐshí	1.5 liǎng
dàhuáng	1 liǎng 18 zhū
lòulú	0.5 liǎng

（一）上十四味，咬咀，以水五升，煮取一升八合。

（二）兒五六歲者，一服四五合。七八歲者，一服六合。

（三）十歲至十四五者，加大黃半兩，足水為一斗，煮取二升半，分三服。

Preparation

(1) Pound the fourteen ingredients above and decoct in 5 *shēng* of water until reduced to 1 *shēng* and 8 *gě*.

(2) For a child of five or six *suì*, one dose should be 4-5 *gě*. For a child of seven or eight *suì*, a dose should be 6 *gě*.

(3) For a child of ten to fourteen or fifteen *suì*, add 0.5 *liǎng* of *dàhuáng* and enough water to make [a total of] 1 *dǒu*. Decoct until reduced to 2.5 *shēng* and divide into three doses.

Commentary VIII.5 ✦ Julian Scott

This symptom picture would (mistakenly) be given the diagnosis erysipelas today. It is quite commonly seen in clinic. Orthodox treatment is with antibiotics, which addresses the momentary outbreak, but the condition just keeps coming back, year after year.

治小兒火灼瘡，一身盡有，如麻豆，或有膿汁，
乍痛乍癢者方。

甘草	
芍藥	
白薟	
黃芩	各半兩
黃連	
黃柏	
苦參	

上七味，末之，以蜜和，敷之，日二夜一。亦可
作湯洗之。

VIII.5.b Unnamed Formula to Treat Wounds from Being Burned by Fire that are Present All Over the Body

Indication

A formula for small children, to treat wounds from being burned by fire that are present all over the body, resemble leprosy, may be purulent, and are alternatingly painful and itching.

Ingredients

gāncǎo	
sháoyào	
báiliǎn	
huángqín	0.5 *liǎng* each
huánglián	
huángbò	
kǔshēn	

Preparation

Pulverize the seven ingredients above and combine with honey. Apply [the mixture to the sores] twice a day and once at night. You can also make a decoction [with the herbs] and wash [the patient] with it.

治小兒瘡初起熛漿似火瘡，名曰熛瘡，亦名爛瘡
方。

（一）桃仁熟搗，以面脂和，敷之。

（二）亦治遍身赤腫起。

又方

馬骨燒灰敷之。

VIII.5.c Unnamed Formula to Treat Blazing Sores

Indication

A formula for small children, to treat sores that begin with blisters rising up, blazing, and a thick fluid,[16] resembling burn sores. These are called blazing sores and are also referred to as festering sores.

Ingredients and Preparation

(1) Thoroughly crush *táorén* and combine with face salve.[17] Apply it [to the sores].

(2) [This formula] also treats redness, swelling, and elevation all over the body.

Another Formula

Char horse bones into ashes and apply [to the sores].

---

16 The concrete meaning of "blazing and a thick fluid" 㶾㮣 is somewhat unclear. The entry on "Black Cinnabar" 黑丹 in vol. 31 of the *Zhū Bìng Yuán Hòu Lùn* might provide some insight, suggesting that the two characters should perhaps not be read as a compound but as two separate symptoms: "Black Cinnabar, when it first erupts, is also [like White Cinnabar] marked by itching and pain, then possibly by blazing, swelling, and elevation, and slightly black color. It is due to complication [of ordinary Cinnabar conditions that are due to wind heat] by wind cold, which causes the blackness (黑丹者，初發亦瘡痛，或㶾腫起，微黑色，由挾風冷，故色黑也。). I consequently interpret "blazing" here as a description of the virulent nature of the sores, which burst forth like raging flames. Alternatively, the "blazing thick fluid" could refer to the highly infectious or irritating nature of the liquid that is oozing from the sores and causing them to spread like a wildfire.

17 This term may be intended here as a generic term, or refer specifically to either of two formulas for "face salve" (面脂) found in Volume 6 of the *Qiān Jīn Fāng*.

水銀膏

治小兒熱瘡方。

水銀	
胡粉	各三兩
松脂	

上三味，以豬脂四升煎松脂，水氣盡，下二物攪令勻，不見水銀，以敷之。

治小兒上下遍身生瘡方。

芍藥	
黃連	各三兩
黃芩	
苦參	八兩
大黃	二兩
蛇床子	一升
黃柏	五兩
菝葜	一斤

上八味　　，咬咀，以水二斗，煮取一斗，以浸浴兒。

VIII.5.d Shuǐyín Gāo (Mercury Salve)

Indication

A formula for small children, to treat heat sores.

Ingredients

shuǐyín	
húfěn	3 *liǎng* each
sōngzhī	

Preparation

Of the three ingredients above, simmer the *sōngzhī* with 4 *shēng* of lard until all moisture has evaporated. Add the other two ingredients and stir until they are evenly mixed in and you cannot see the *shuǐyín*. Spread this [on the sores].

VIII.5.e Unnamed Formula

Indication

A formula for small children, to treat the formation of sores on both the upper and lower body and all over the body.

Ingredients

sháoyào	
huánglián	3 *liǎng* each
huángqín	
kǔshēn	8 *liǎng*
dàhuáng	2 *liǎng*
shéchuángzǐ	1 *shēng*
huángbò	5 *liǎng*
báqiā	1 *jīn*

Preparation

Pound the eight ingredients above and decoct in 2 *dǒu* of water until reduced to 1 *dǒu*. Use this to bathe the child.

苦參湯

浴小兒身上下百瘡不瘥方。

苦參	八兩
地榆	
黃連	
王不留行	各三兩
獨活	
艾葉	
竹葉	二升

上七味，㕮咀，以水三斗，煮取一斗，以浴兒瘡上。浴訖，敷黃連散。

VIII.5.f Kǔshēn Tāng (Flavescent Sophora Decoction)

Indication

A formula for bathing small children who have a hundred sores up and down their body that will not heal.

Ingredients

kǔshēn	8 *liǎng*
dìyú	3 *liǎng* each
huánglián	
wángbùliúxíng	
dúhuó	
àiyè	
zhúyè	2 *shēng*

Preparation

Pound the seven ingredients above and decoct in 3 *dǒu* of water until reduced to 1 *dǒu*. Use this as a wash on the child's sores. When you are finished with the wash, apply Huánglián Sǎn.

治三日小兒頭面瘡起，身體大熱方。

升麻	
柴胡	各六銖
石膏	
甘草	各十二銖
當歸	
大黃	各十八銖
黃芩	

（一）上七味，㕮咀，以水四升，煮取二升，分
　　　服。日三夜一。

（二）量兒大小用之。

治小兒身體、頭面悉生瘡方。

（一）榆白皮隨多少，曝令燥，下篩，醋和塗綿
　　　以敷瘡上，蟲自出。

（二）亦可以豬脂和塗之。

VIII.5.g Unnamed Formula for Three-day-old Children, to Treat Sores that Rise Up on the Head and Face, with Great Heat in the Body

Ingredients

shēngmá	6 *zhū* each
cháihú	
shígāo	
gāncǎo	12 *zhū* each
dāngguī	
dàhuáng	18 *zhū* each
huángqín	

Preparation

(1) Pound the seven ingredients above and decoct in 4 *shēng* of water until reduced to 2 *shēng*. Divide into doses. [Give] three doses during the day and one at night.

(2) Use in accordance with the child's size.

VIII.5.h Unnamed Formula to Treat the Formation of Sores Everywhere on the Body and on the Head and Face

Indication

A formula for small children, to treat the formation of sores everywhere on the body and on the head and face.

Ingredients and Preparation

(1) Take an appropriate amount of *yúbáipí* and leave it out in the sun to dry. Sift it, mix it with vinegar, and spread it on silk floss. Use this to apply it to the sores. The worms will come out on their own.

(2) You can also mix it with lard and spread it on [as a salve].

《衍義》

（一）五香枳實湯與五香連翹湯大同小異。

（二）彼以毒腫色白，且有惡核瘰癧，故用連翹、海藻、射乾、竹瀝軟堅滌痰之品以輔五香。

（三）此治風熱(疒音)瘭堅如麻豆，故用防風、秦艽、白蘞、漏蘆透風利竅之品以輔五香，各隨佐使應用。

（四）其小兒火灼瘡，一身盡如麻豆，用芩、連、黃柏，專治熱毒。

（五）白蘞、苦參散結止痛。

（六）白芍、甘草解毒和營。

（七）小兒上下遍身生瘡，即於前方除去白蘞、甘草加大黃，以合三黃。

（八）並入蛇床、撥葜以除痺濕之毒。

Yǎn Yì (Expanded Meaning)

(1) Wǔ Xiāng Zhǐshí Tāng and Wǔxiāng Liánqiáo Tāng are basically identical with minor differences.

(2) The latter addresses the presence of toxic swelling with a white complexion as well as the presence of malign nodules and scrofula. Therefore it uses *liánqiáo, hǎizǎo, shègān*, and *zhúlì*, which are substances that soften hardenings and sweep away phlegm, to assist the five fragrances.

(3) The former treats wind heat with dormant papules that are hard and resemble leprosy. Therefore it uses *fángfēng, qínjiāo, báiliǎn*, and *lòulú*, which are all substances that outthrust wind and disinhibit the orifices, to assist the five fragrances. Each formula should be used in accordance with its ministers and envoys.

(4) The treatment for wounds from being burned by fire that are present all over the body and resemble leprosy in small children uses *huángqín, huánglián*, and *huángbò* to specifically treat heat toxin.

(5) *Báiliǎn* and *kǔshēn* dissipate binds and relieve pain.

(6) *Báisháo* and *gāncǎo* resolve toxin and harmonize *yíng* construction.

(7) In comparison with the preceding formula, the formula to treat the formation of sores on both the upper and lower body and all over the body in small children has eliminated *báiliǎn* and *gāncǎo* but added *dàhuáng*, to join the three "*huáng*."[18]

(8) At the same time, it has added *shéchuángzǐ* and *báqiā* to eliminate the toxins of impediment dampness.

---

18 "Three *huáng*" is a reference to the other three ingredients with the character 黄 in their names, namely *huánglián, huángqín*, and *huángbò*.

（九）其桃仁和面脂專取散血之用。

（十）馬骨燒灰祛風止痛，活血舒筋。

（十一）水銀、胡粉、松脂熬豬脂傅，專行燥濕。

（十二）苦參浴兒，專取苦燥以治濕熱。

（十三）三日小兒胎毒炘發，頭面瘡起，身體大熱，故用石膏、大黃、黃芩引導毒從下泄。

（十四）升麻、柴胡乘機外分其勢，當歸、甘草和其始生血氣也。

（十五）榆白皮性滑利竅，得醋或豬脂和塗，能使瘡中之蟲自出。

(9) The formula for *táorén* mixed with face salve specifically utilizes its effect of dissipating blood.

(10) Horse bones charred into ashes dispel wind and relieve pain, enliven blood and soothe the sinews.

(11) *Shuǐyín*, *húfěn*, and *sōngzhī*, when simmered in lard and applied [to the affected area], specifically act to dry up dampness.

(12) Washing the child with *kǔshēn* specifically takes advantage of its bitter dryness to treat damp heat.

(13) To treat a three-day-old baby who is suffering from fetal toxin flaming up, which manifests with sores rising up on the head and face accompanied by great heat in the body, we therefore use *shígāo*, *dàhuáng*, and *huángqín* to draw the toxin out by draining it from the lower body.

(14) *Shēngmá* and *cháihú* seize the opportunity to externally divide their might, while *dāngguī* and *gāncǎo* harmonize the patient's beginning production of blood and qì.

(15) *Yúbáipí* is by nature slippery and disinhibits the orifices. When combined with vinegar or lard and spread on the body, it is able to cause the worms in any sores to exit spontaneously.

枳實丸

（一）治小兒病風瘙，癢痛如疥，搔之汁出，遍身(疒广音)瘡如麻豆粒，年年喜發，面目虛肥，手足乾枯，毛髮細黃，及肌膚不光澤，鼻氣不利。

（二）此則少時熱盛極，體當風，風熱相搏所得也。不早治之，成大風疾方。

枳實	一兩半
菊花	
蛇床子	
防風	
白薇	各一兩
浮萍	
蒺藜子	
天雄	
麻黃	各半兩
漏蘆	

VIII.6 Zhǐshí Wán (Unripe Bitter Orange Pills)

Indication

(1) A formula for small children, to treat conditions of wind itch, with itching and pain that resemble scabies, liquid coming out when the sores are scratched, dormant papules all over the body that resemble leprosy, and a tendency for the condition to erupt year after year. This is accompanied by a vacuous and greasy face and eyes, withered dry hands and feet, fine yellowish body hair and hair on the head, as well as lusterless skin and nasal congestion.[19]

(2) This [condition] results from heat that reached an extreme state of exuberance in early childhood and was further complicated when the body has been exposed to wind, so that wind and heat are now struggling with each other. If you do not treat this early on, it turns into a serious wind disease.

Ingredients

zhǐshí	1.5 *liǎng*
júhuā	1 *liǎng* each
shéchuángzǐ	
fángfēng	
báiwēi	
fúpíng	
jílízǐ	
tiānxióng	0.5 *liǎng* each
máhuáng	
lòulú	

---

19 鼻氣不利 *bí qì bú lì*: Literally, "inhibited nose qì."

（一）上十味，末之，蜜和如大豆許。

（二）五歲兒飲服十丸，加至二十丸，日二。

（三）五歲以上者，隨意加之。兒大者可為散
　　　服。

枳實丸《衍義》

（一）方中浮萍、麻黃、防風、刺蒺藜、菊花、
　　　白薇，專祛風毒外泄。

（二）枳實、漏蘆，專祛風內泄。

（三）天雄、蛇床，專祛經絡中風毒，不使伏藏
　　　而成惡疾也。

Preparation

(1) Pulverize the ten ingredients above and mix with honey [into pills] about the size of soybeans.

(2) For a child of five *suì*, give ten pills per dose in liquid, increasing the dosage up to twenty pills, twice a day.

(3) For a patient older than five *suì*, increase the dosage at your discretion. An older child can also take this formula as a powder.

Zhǐshí Wán (Unripe Bitter Orange Pills) *Yǎn Yì* (Expanded Meaning)

(1) The *fúpíng, máhuáng, fángfēng, jílízǐ, júhuā,* and *báiwēi* in this formula specifically dispel wind toxin by draining it externally.

(2) The *zhǐshí* and *lòulú* specifically dispel wind by draining it internally.

(3) The *tiānxióng* and *shéchuángzǐ* specifically dispel the wind toxin from the channels and network vessels, preventing it from going into hiding deep down and forming malign diseases [later on].

治小兒風瘙癮疹方。

蒴藋	
防風	
羊桃	
石楠	
秦椒	
升麻	
苦參	各一兩
茵芋	
芫花	
蒺藜	
蛇床子	
枳實	
礬石	

上十三味，㕮咀，以漿水三斗，煮取一斗，去
滓，納礬，令小沸，浴之。

VIII.7 Formulas for Wind Itch and Dormant Papules[20]

Ingredients

shuòdiào	
fángfēng	
yángtáo	
shínán	
qínjiāo	
shēngmá	
kǔshēn	1 *liǎng* each
yīnyù	
*yuánhuā**	
jílì	
shéchuángzǐ	
zhǐshí	
fánshí	

*Editorial comment: Another edition has *chōngwèi* instead.

Preparation

Of the thirteen ingredients above, pound [everything but the *fánshí*] and decoct in 3 *dǒu* of sour millet water until reduced to 1 *dǒu*. Remove the dregs, add the *fánshí*, and bring to a small boil. Wash [the patient] with this.

---

20 This indication is most likely equivalent to the biomedical condition of urticaria.

《衍義》

（一）方下雖治風瘙癮疹，與前方主治不殊。

（二）方中除枳實、蛇床、防風、蒺藜四味相
　　　同，其蒴藋、羊桃、石南、苦參、茵芋、
　　　芫花皆毒風痹濕拘攣藥。

（三）惟秦椒、升麻升散熱邪，礜石收斂濕熱。

（四）豈特專主方下諸治哉。

Yǎn Yì (Expanded Meaning)

(1) Even though the present formula states that it treats wind itch and dormant papules, its indications are no different than those of the previous formula.

(2) In addition to the four ingredients zhǐshí, shéchuángzǐ, fángfēng, and jílì, which are identical with the preceding formula, the shuòdiào, yángtáo, shínán, kǔshēn, yínyù, and yuánhuā here are all medicinals for toxic wind, bì impediment-type dampness, and hypertonicity.

(3) Only qínjiāo and shēngmá raise and dissipate heat evil, while fánshí astringes damp heat.

(4) How could you limit yourself specifically to the indication of each formula when administering the various treatments?

又方:

（一）牛膝末，酒服方寸匕。

（二）漏瘡多年不瘥，搗末敷之。亦主骨疽、癲疾、瘰癧，絕妙。

《衍義》

（一）牛膝專行筋脈。

（二）《本經》治寒濕痿痹，四肢拘攣，膝痛不可屈伸。

（三）《千金》治漏瘡多年不瘥，及骨疽癲疾瘰癧。

（四）非取其走肝榮筋之力歟。

VIII.8 Formula for Fistulas

(1) Pulverize *niúxī* and take a square-*cùn* spoon in liquor.

(2) For fistulas that have not healed for many years, crush and pulverize [*niúxī*] and spread it on [the affected area]. This formula also rules bone flat-abscesses, withdrawal disease, and scrofula. It is of utmost ingenuity.

Yǎn Yì (Expanded Meaning)

(1) *Niúxī* specifically acts on the sinews and vessels.

(2) According to the *Shénnóng Běncǎo Jīng*, it treats cold- and damp-type wilting and *bì* impediment, hypertonicity of the limbs, and knee pain [so severe that the patient] is unable to bend or stretch [the knee].

(3) According to the *Qiān Jīn Fāng*, it treats fistulas that have not healed for many years as well as bone flat-abscesses, withdrawal disease, and scrofula.

(4) How could this not be a case of taking advantage of its power to penetrate the liver and make the sinews thrive?

澤蘭湯

主丹及癮疹入腹殺人方。

澤蘭	
芎藭	
附子	
茵芋	各十二銖
藁本	
莽草	
細辛	

（一）上七味，㕮咀，以水三升，煮取一升半。
　　　分四服。

（二）先服此湯，然後作餘治。

《衍義》

（一）一切浮腫，總是氣虛溫熱。

（二）此用小便溫漬，專解蘊蒸熱毒。

VIII.9 Zélán Tāng (Lycopus Decoction)

Indication

A formula that rules cinnabar [toxin] as well as dormant papules, which will kill the patient once the condition enters the abdomen.

Ingredients

zélán	
xiōngqióng	
fùzǐ	
yīnyù	12 *zhū* each
gǎoběn	
mǎngcǎo	
xìxīn	

Preparation

(1) Pound the seven ingredients above and decoct in 3 *shēng* of water until reduced to 1.5 *shēng*. Divide into four doses.

(2) First take this decoction and then afterwards apply additional treatments.[21]

21　On the basis of the *Yǎn Yì* commentary, this appears to be referring to the following treatment of soaking the swollen limbs in urine. I have purposely left it more literal, though, because that is merely the interpretation provided by Zhāng Lù but not necessarily the only possible reading of this line.

Yǎn Yì (Expanded Meaning)

(1) Every single case of superficial swelling is always [related to] qì vacuity with warmth or heat.

(2) The present [treatment plan] uses urine as a warm soak to specifically resolve the smoldering and steaming heat toxin.

治小兒手足及身腫方。

以小便溫暖漬之，良。

又方

巴豆五十枚，去心皮，以水三升，煮取一升，以綿內湯中，拭病上，隨手消。並治癮疹。

論曰

（一）小兒頭生小瘡，浸淫疽癢，黃膏出，不生痂，連年不差者，亦名妒頭瘡。

（二）以赤龍皮湯及天麻湯洗之。

（三）內服漏蘆湯，外宜敷飛烏膏散，及黃連胡粉水銀膏散。

VIII.10 Formulas for Swelling

VIII.10a Unnamed Formula for Small Children, to Treat Swelling in the Hands and Feet as well as Generalized Swelling

Taking urine, warming it up, and soaking [the swollen part of the body] in it is excellent.

Another Formula

Take 50 pieces of *bādòu* and remove the skin of the seed. Decoct in 3 *shēng* of water until reduced to 1 *shēng*. Put some silk floss in the decoction and then wipe this on top of the disease[d area]. [The swelling] will disperse right along with your wiping. This [formula] also treats dormant papules.

VIII.11 Essay

(1) When small children form small sores on the head that are moist, spreading, flat-abscessed, and itching, with a yellow paste[-like substance] coming out, and fail to form a scab or heal for year after year, [this condition] is also called "jealous head sores."

(2) Wash them with Chìlóngpí Tāng (Mongolian Oak Bark Decoction) and Tiānmá Tāng (Gastrodia Decoction).

(3) Internally take Lòulú Tāng. Externally, it is recommended to apply Fēiwū Gāo Sǎn (Flying Black Paste Powder) as well as Huánglián Húfěn Shuǐyíngāo Sǎn (Coptis, Processed Galenite, and Mercury Paste Powder).[22]

---

22 The formula for Lòulú Tāng is the first formula in this chapter. See above, p. 231. The other formulas are all found in volume 23, in the second section on "Intestinal Ulcers" (腸癰 *cháng yōng*). They appear to be primarily indicated for breast sores and various other oozing sores, men's genital sores, erosion-type sores, etc. The name "Flying Black" presumably refers to the first ingredient, which is the condensation of black smoke rising from roasting cinnabar in the production of liquid mercury. In combination with alum (礬石 *fánshí*), this constitutes the Flying Black Paste or Powder Formula, which is applied as a paste or powder to the sore on the breast or elsewhere. The first two formulas consist of decoctions made by simmering chopped Mongolian oak bark and gastrodia rhizome, respectively, which are applied warm or cool, as comfortable, to the breast sore or other chronic festering sores.

藜蘆膏

治小兒一切頭瘡，久即疽癢不生痂方。

藜蘆	各二兩
黃連	
雄黃	
黃芩	
松脂	
豬脂	半斤
礬石	五兩

（一）上七味，末之，煎令調和。

（二）先以赤龍皮天麻湯洗訖，敷之。

VIII.12 Formulas for Chronic Head Sores

VIII.12.a Lílú Gāo (Veratrum Salve)

Indication

A formula for small children, to treat all head sores that have become chronic and then turned into flat-abscesses that itch and fail to form scabs.

Ingredients

lílú	
huánglián	
xiónghuáng	2 *liǎng* each
huángqín	
sōngzhī*	
zhūzhī	0.5 *jīn*
fánshí	5 *liǎng*

*Translator's note: Some editions have 3 *liǎng* here instead.

Preparation

(1) Of the seven ingredients above, pulverize the dry ones and simmer everything until they are combined well.

(2) After you have first finished washing [the sores] with Chìlóngpí Tāng and Tiānmá Tāng, apply [this salve].[23]

---

23   See the previous note and *Qiān Jīn Fāng* volume 23, section 2 for information about these formulas.

治小兒頭瘡經年不瘥方。

松脂	
苦參	各一兩半
黃連	
大黃	各一兩
胡粉	
黃芩	各一兩六銖
水銀	
礬石	半兩
蛇床子	十八銖

上九味，末之，以臘月豬脂和，研水銀不見，敷
之。

又方
取屋塵末和油瓶下滓，以皂莢湯洗，敷之。

又方
取大蟲脂敷之。亦治白禿。

又方
髮中生瘡頂白者，皆以熊白敷之。

VIII.12.b Additional Formulas for Sores on the Head

Formula for small children, to treat sores on the head that have failed to heal for several years in a row.

Ingredients

sōngzhī	
kǔshēn	1.5 *liǎng* each
huánglián	
dàhuáng	
húfěn	1 *liǎng* each
huángqín	
shuǐyín	1 *liǎng* 6 *zhū* each
fánshí	0.5 *liǎng*
shéchuángzǐ	18 *zhū*

Preparation

Of the nine ingredients above, pulverize [all the dry ingredients] and combine everything with lard from the twelfth lunar month. Grind in the *shuǐyín* until you can no longer see it. Apply this [to the sores].

Another Formula

Take house dust, pulverize it, and combine it with the dregs from the bottom of an oil bottle. Wash [the sores] with Zàojiá Tāng (Gleditsia Decoction) and then apply this formula.

Another Formula

Take tiger fat and apply it [to the sores]. This also treats white hair and baldness.

Another Formula

When there are white-tipped sores forming in the hair on the head, in all cases spread white bear fat[24] on them.

---

24 As Táo Hóngjǐng explains (cited in the *Běncǎo Gāngmù*), this is the fat from the bear's back, which is white like jade in color, is most delicious in flavor, and can only be obtained in the winter months

治小兒頭瘡方。

胡粉	一兩
黃連	二兩

上二味，末之，洗瘡去痂，拭乾，敷之即瘥。更發，如前敷之。

又方

胡粉	各一兩
連翹	
水銀	半兩

上三味，以水煎連翹，納胡粉、水銀和調，敷之。

又方

胡粉	各二兩
白松脂	
水銀	一兩
豬脂	四兩

上四味合煎，去滓，納水銀粉，調敷之。大人患同。

Unnamed formula

For small children, to treat sores on the head.

Ingredients

húfěn	1 *liǎng*
huánglián	2 *liǎng*

Preparation

Pulverize the two ingredients above. Wash the sores and remove any scabs. Wipe them dry. Applying [this powder] causes immediate healing. If they erupt again, apply it as before.

Another Formula

Ingredients

húfěn	1 *liǎng* each
liánqiáo	
shuǐyín	0.5 *liǎng*

Preparation

Of the three ingredients above, simmer the *liánqiáo* in water and then add the *húfěn* and *shuǐyín*, mixing them until well blended. Apply this [to the sores].

Another Formula

Ingredients

húfěn	2 *liǎng* each
báisōngzhī	
shuǐyín	1 *liǎng*
zhūzhī	4 *liǎng*

Preparation

Of the four ingredients above, simmer [everything except for the *shuǐyín*] together. Remove the dregs, add the pulverized *shuǐyín*, and mix it well. Apply this [to the sores]. The treatment for adults suffering from this condition is identical.

《衍義》

（一）藜蘆吐風痰藥，兼芩、連燥濕，雄黃解
　　　莓，礬石、松脂以收濕熱。

（二）赤龍皮煎湯洗，除蟲及漏惡瘡。

（三）天麻療蠱毒惡風，為治風毒要藥。

（四）其治小兒頭瘡經年不瘥方，即前方去藜
　　　蘆、雄黃，加大黃、苦參、蛇床子、胡
　　　粉、水銀等，皆袪濕熱之藥。

（五）屋塵油滓腐穢之物，取治腐穢之疾。

（六）熊脂逐風，專治頭瘍白禿，面上皯皰。

（七）胡粉、黃連，胡粉、連翹、水銀，胡粉、
　　　水銀、松脂、豬脂總傅小兒頭瘡，咸取殺
　　　蟲燥濕之義。

Yăn Yì (Expanded Meaning)

(1) *Lílú* is a medicinal that "vomits out" wind and phlegm. It is combined [in the formula here] with *huángqín* and *huánglián*, which dry dampness, *xiónghuáng*, which resolves toxin, and with *fánshí* and *sōngzhī* to astringe damp heat.

(2) Washing [the head sores] with *chìlóngpí* brewed into a decoction gets rid of the worms and of leaking and malign sores.

(3) *Tiānmá* cures *gŭ* toxin and malign wind and is a crucial medicinal for treating wind toxin.

(4) The formula here for treating "small children's sores on the head that have failed to heal for several years in a row" is identical to the previous formula, but without *lílú* and *xiónghuáng*, and with *dàhuáng, kŭshēn, shéchuángzĭ, húfěn*, and *shuǐyín* added, all of which are medicinals for dispelling damp heat.

(5) House dust and oil dregs are rotten and filthy substances. They are here used to treat rotten and filthy conditions.

(6) Bear fat expels wind and specifically treats festering sores on the head, white hair and baldness, and pimples in the face.

(7) The combinations of *húfěn* and *huánglián*; of *húfěn, liánqiáo*, and *shuǐyín*; and of *húfěn, shuǐyín, sōngzhī*, and *zhūzhī* all specifically treat small children's head sores. Their saltiness has the significance of killing worms and drying dampness.

苦參洗湯

治小兒頭瘡方。

苦參	
黃芩	
黃連	
黃柏	各一兩
甘草	
大黃	
芎藭	
蒺藜子	三合

上八味，咬咀，以水六升，煮取三升，漬布搨瘡上，日數過。

《衍義》

（一）芩、連、大黃、黃柏、苦參等一派苦寒藥中。

（二）但得川芎一味和血，蒺藜一味透風，甘草一味解毒。

（三）煎湯漬布頻拓瘡上，自愈。

VIII.13 Kǔshēn Xǐ Tāng (Flavescent Sophora Wash Decoction)

Indication
A formula for small children, to treat head sores.

Ingredients

kǔshēn	
huángqín	
huánglián	
huángbò	1 *liǎng* each
gāncǎo	
dàhuáng	
xiōngqióng	
jílízǐ	3 *gě*

Preparation
Pound the eight ingredients above and decoct in 6 *shēng* of water until reduced to 3 *shēng*. Soak a cloth [in the decoction] and rub it on the sores, several times a day.

Yǎn Yì (Expanded Meaning)

(1) *Huángqín, huánglián, dàhuáng, huángbò,* and *kǔshēn* all belong to the category of bitter cold medicinals.

(2) The formula only contains the single ingredient *chuānxiōng* for harmonizing the blood, the single ingredient *jílì* for outthrusting wind, and the single ingredient *gāncǎo* for resolving toxin.

(3) Simmering the ingredients into a decoction, soaking a cloth in this preparation, and then rubbing this cloth repeatedly on the sores results in spontaneous recovery.

治小兒頭上惡毒腫痤癤諸瘡方。

（一）男子屎尖燒灰，和臘月豬脂。
（二）先以醋泔清淨洗，拭乾，敷之。

治小兒禿頭瘡方。

取雄雞屎，陳醬、苦酒和，以洗瘡了，敷之。

又方

芫花，臘月豬脂和如泥，洗去痂。拭乾，敷之，日一度。

治小兒頭禿瘡方

葶藶子細末，先洗，敷之。

又方
不中水蕪菁葉燒作灰，和豬脂敷之。

VIII.14 Formulas for Sores, Baldness, & Fistulas

VIII.14.a Formula for All Kinds of Sores with Malign Toxin, Swelling, Acne, and Boils on the Head

Ingredients and Preparation

(1) Take a pointed piece of excrement from a male adult or child[25] and char it into ashes. Mix this with lard from the twelfth lunar month.

(2) First clean and wash [the sores] with soured rice-washing liquid and wipe them dry. Then apply this [salve].

VIII.14.b Formulas for Baldness and Sores on the Head

Take excrement from a rooster, old pickling liquid, and bitter liquor. Blend [the liquids] together and use this to wash the sores. Afterwards spread on [the rooster droppings].[26]

Another Formula

Blend *yuánhuā* and lard from the twelfth lunar month into a mud-like consistency. Wash [the sores] and remove any scabs. Wipe [the area] dry and apply [this formula], once a day.

Another Formula

Process *tínglìzǐ* into a fine powder. First wash [the sores] and then apply this.

Another Formula

Take turnip leaves that have not been put into water and char them into ashes. Blend with lard and spread it on [the sores].

VIII.14.c Unnamed Formula for Small Children, to Treat

---

25 男子 *nán zǐ*: This term can mean either "male adult" or "male child" - either meaning is already found in early texts, so it is unclear here which of the two this particular formula refers to.

26 The grammatical structure of this sentence is not clear, and the three ingredients are just listed in a row. My reading is based strictly on an effort to make clinical sense of it.

治小兒頭禿瘡，無髮苦癢方。

野葛末	
豬脂	各一兩
羊脂	

上三味，合煎令消，待冷，以敷之，不過三上。

一物楸葉方

治少兒頭不生髮方。

楸葉搗取汁，敷頭上，立生。

Baldness and Sores on the Head, Lack of Head Hair, Soreness, and Itching.

Ingredients

yěgé, pulverized	
lard	1 *liǎng* each
mutton fat	

Preparation

Blend the three ingredients above and simmer, causing them to dissolve. Wait until [the mixture] has cooled off and then spread it on. Do not exceed three applications.

VIII.14.d Yī Wù Qiūyè Fāng (Single-Ingredient Manchurian Catalpa Formula)

Indication

A formula for youth,[27] to treat failure to grow hair on the head.

Ingredients and Preparation

Pound *qiūyè* to obtain the juice. Apply this to the top of the head, and the hair will immediately start growing.

VIII.14.e Unnamed Formula for Small Children, to Treat

---

27   It is unclear to me whether the term 少兒 *shào ér* here is an error or an intentional deviation from the norm. All the other formulas for pediatrics in this chapter address conditions of "small children" (小兒 *xiǎo ér*), which is almost the same character with only one more stroke added. The compound 少兒 is not commonly used in classical sources and is not found anywhere else in the *Qiān Jīn Fāng*. The compound 少小 *shào xiǎo* does occur occasionally. I have translated that term as "children" or "childhood" – as opposed to the more specific "small children" for 小兒. *Shào xiǎo* is often used in medical literature to refer to pediatric conditions.

治小兒頭不生髮方。

燒鯽魚灰末，以醬汁和，敷之。

治小兒瘻瘡方。

冢中石灰敷之，厚著之良。

又方
燒桑根灰敷之，並燒烏羊角作灰，相和敷之。

治小兒疽瘻方。

丹砂	三十銖
雄黃	二十四銖
礜石	十八銖，馬齒者
雌黃	二十四銖
大黃	三十銖
黃連	三十六銖
莽草	十八銖
⊠茹	二十四銖，漆頭者

Failure to Grow Hair on the Head

Char golden carp into ashes and pulverize. Blend it with pickling liquid and spread it on.

VIII.14.f Unnamed Formulas for Small Children, to Treat Fistulas

Spread lime from inside a tomb on [the fistula]. Applying it thickly is excellent.

Another formula

Char *sānggén* into ashes and spread that on [the fistula]. Also, char a black sheep or goat's horn into ashes, mix it with [the charred *sānggén*], and apply that.

VIII.14.g Unnamed Formula for Small Children, to Treat Flat-abscessed Fistula

Ingredients

dānshā	30 *zhū*
xiónghuáng	24 *zhū*
fánshí	18 *zhū* (unprocessed)
cíhuáng	24 *zhū*
dàhuáng	30 *zhū*
huánglián	36 *zhū*
mǎngcǎo	18 *zhū*
lúrú	24 *zhū* (the highest grade)

Preparation

（一）上八味，咬咀，以豬脂一升三合，微火煎三上三下。

（二）膏成，去滓，下諸石末攪凝，敷之。

治小兒惡瘡方。

熬豉令黃，末之，敷瘡上，不過三敷愈。

治小兒疸極，月初即生，常有黃水出方。

（一）醋和油煎令如粥及熱，敷之，二日一易。

（二）欲重敷，則以皂莢湯洗瘡，仍敷之。

(1) Of the eight ingredients above, pound [the herbs] and simmer in 1 *shēng* and 3 *gě* of lard over a small flame, bringing [the mixture] to a boil three times.

(2) When the paste is done, remove the dregs, add the various minerals as powders and stir until it thickens. Spread this on [the fistula].

VIII.14.h Unnamed Formula for Small Children, to Treat Malign Sores

Toast *dòuchǐ* until yellow, pulverize it, and apply it on top of the sore. No more than three applications will result in recovery.[28]

VIII.14.i Unnamed Formula for Small Children, to Treat Extreme Cases of Flat-abscesses that Form Right at the Beginning of the [Lunar] Month and Constantly have a Yellow Discharge

(1) Simmer vinegar and oil until it has reached a gruel-like consistency and is hot. Spread it on, changing the dressing once every two days.

(2) If you want to apply it again, first wash the sore with Zàojiá Tāng and then spread it on.

VIII.14.j Unnamed Formula for Small Children, to Treat Lunar

---

28 In strictly grammatical terms, it is also possible to read this last phrase, 不過三敷愈, as "Do not exceed three applications, and recovery [will ensue]." Given the innocuous nature of the single ingredient *dòuchǐ*, however, this interpretation is less likely.

治小兒月蝕瘡，隨月生死方。

以胡粉和酥敷之，五日瘥。

治月蝕，九竅皆有瘡方：

燒蚯蚓屎末，和豬膏敷之。

又方
水和粉敷之。

Erosion Sores,[29] which Appear and Disappear in Conjunction with the Moon

Mix *húfěn* with butter and spread it on [the sores]. After five days, the patient is cured.

VIII.14.k Unnamed Formulas to treat Lunar Erosion [Sores] that Affect All Nine Orifices

Char earthworm excrement and pulverize it. Mix it with lard and spread it on.

Another Formula

Mix water with rice flour and spread it on [the sores].

VIII.14.l Unnamed Formula for Small Children, to Treat Moist

---

29 月蝕瘡 *yùe shí chuāng*: According to the *Zhū Bìng Yuán Hòu Lùn* (vol. 35, chapter 30 on "Eclipse Sores"), the condition describes "sores that form around the ears and nose of small children and are called such because they grow and shrink in accordance with the moon. People say that when babies look at the moon when it is new and point at it with a finger, this causes them to form sores below the ears." 小兒耳鼻口間生瘡，世謂之月食瘡，隨月生死，因以為名也。世云小兒見月初生，以手指指之，則令耳下生瘡，故呼為月食瘡也。

治小兒浸淫瘡方。

灶中黃土
髮灰

上二味，各等分，末之，以豬脂和敷之。

治小兒黃爛瘡方。

四交道中土
灶下土

上二味，各等分，末之以敷。

又方
燒艾灰敷之。

又方
燒牛屎敷之。亦滅瘢。

Spreading Sores

Ingredients

zàozhōnghuángtǔ (oven earth)
fàhuī (ashed hair)

Preparation

Take equal amounts of the two ingredients above and pulverize them. Mix with lard and spread it on.

VIII.14.m Unnamed Formula for Small Children, to Treat Yellow Putrefying Sores

Ingredients

dirt from the middle of a four-way intersection
dirt from underneath the stove

Preparation

Take equal amounts of the two ingredients above and pulverize them. Spread [the mixture] on [the sores].[30]

Another Formula

Char *àiyè* into ashes and spread it on.

Another Formula

Char cow manure and spread it on. [This treatment] also causes scars to vanish.

VIII.14.l Unnamed Formulas to Treat Scabies

---

30 Editorial comment: This also treats crying at night.

治小兒疥方。

燒竹葉為灰，雞子白和敷之，日三。亦治(瘑)瘡。

又方
燒亂髮灰，和臘月豬脂，敷之。

又方
以臭酥和胡粉，敷之。

治小兒頭面瘡疥方。
麻子五升，末之，以水和，絞取汁，與蜜和，敷之。若有白犬膽敷之，大佳。

Char *zhúyè* into ashes. Mix with egg whites and spread it on, three times a day. [This formula] also treats baldness and sores.[31]

Another Formula

Char *luànfà* into ashes and mix with lard from the twelfth lunar month. Spread it on.

Another Formula

Take rancid butter and mix it with *húfěn*. Spread it on.

Another Formula

Pulverize 5 *shēng* of *mázǐ* and mix with water. Wring it out to get the juice[32] and mix it with honey. Spread this on. If you have white dog bile available, spreading this on [the sores as well] is most excellent.

VIII.14.m Unnamed Formulas to Treat Damp Ringworm

---

31 According to the *Dai Kanwa Jiten* 大漢和辞典 ("Great Dictionary from Chinese to Japanese"), the character (瘯) is very rare and can be either a synonym for 瘡 *chuāng* "sores" or for 禿 *tū* "baldness."

32 Given the fact that the amount of water to use is not specified, it is also possible to read the sentence instead as instructing the practitioner to get rid of the liquid (reading 取汁 as "take the juice" [away]) and use the left-over ground *mázǐ* to mix with the honey. That is less likely though when we consider that 取 "to take" usually has the connotation "to obtain," "to gain."

治小兒濕癬方。

枸杞根搗作末，和臘月豬脂，敷之。

又方
桃青皮搗末，和醋敷之，日二。

又方
揩破，以牛鼻上津敷之。

又方
煎馬尿洗之。

又方
燒狗屎灰，和豬脂塗之。

Pound and pulverize *gǒuqǐgēn*. Mix with lard from the twelfth lunar month and spread it on.

Pound and pulverize green walnut peel[33] and mix with vinegar. Spread it on, twice a day.

Another Formula
Wipe and break [the sores]. Take the saliva from an ox nose and spread it on.

Another Formula
Simmer horse urine and wash [the sores] with it.

Another Formula
Char dog excrement into ashes and mix with lard. Spread it on.

VIII.14.n Unnamed Formula for Small Children, to Treat the

---

33   On the basis of clinical meaning and the expanded explanation in the *Yǎn Yì* translated below, I follow Zhāng Lù in reading 桃 *táo* here as an abbreviation for 核桃 *hé táo* "walnut," also called 胡桃 *hú táo*, instead of as "peach." Black walnut extract is a common ingredient in Western herbalism, and walnut peel (or specifically, the oil extracted by pressure) is also used in Chinese medicine for such purposes as blackening mustaches (when combined in equal parts with tadpoles) or clothing, or treating wind-related skin conditions.

治小兒身上生赤疵方。

取馬尿洗之，日四五度。

治小兒身上有赤黑疵方。

針父腳中，取血貼疵上，即消。

又方
取狗熱屎敷之，皮自卷落。

治小兒疣目方。

以針及小刀子決目四面，令似血出。取患瘡人瘡中汁、黃膿敷之，莫近水三日，即膿潰根動自脫落。

Formation of Red Blemishes on the Body

Take horse urine and wash [the patient's body] with this, four to five times a day.

VIII.14.o Unnamed Formula for Small Children, to Treat the Presence of Red and Black Blemishes on the Body

Prick the center of the father's foot with a needle. Take the blood and paste it on the blemish. [The blemish] will vanish immediately.

Another Formula

Take a dog's hot urine and spread it on [the blemishes]. The skin will peel and drop off on its own.

VIII.14.p Unnamed Formula for Small Children, to Treat Warts[34]

With a needle or a small knife, cut open the wart on all four sides until it looks like blood is coming out. Take the liquid and yellow pus from inside the sore of a person suffering from sores[35] and spread it on. Do not go anywhere near water for three days. Then the pus will burst out and the root will move and drop off spontaneously.

---

34   According to the *Zhū Bìng Yuán Hòu Lùn* (vo. 31, chap. 8 on "Warts"), "Warts are [lesions] that suddenly form on the side of a person's hands or feet, resembling beans or knotted sinews, whether five or ten, connected to each other inside the skin, with a coarse rigid [area] in the flesh. These are also formed as the result of wind evil striking the skin and flesh and transforming (疣目者，人手足邊忽生如豆，或如結筋，或五箇，或十箇，相連肌裏，粗強於 肉，謂之疣目。此亦是風邪搏於肌肉而變生也。)."

35   Grammatically, it is impossible to determine whether "sore" here refers specifically to "warts" and whether the treatment instructs us to use the discharge from another wart from the same patient or from a random sore or another wart from a different person who just happens to be suffering from sores.

《衍義》

（一）雄雞屎下氣殺蟲，以醬醋引入蟲口。

（二）芫花解毒殺蟲，以豬脂引入蟲口。

（三）葶藶破堅利水殺蟲，與芫花不殊。

（四）蕪菁治熱毒風腫。

（五）野葛治惡風水腫殺蟲，以毒攻毒也。

（六）楸葉拔毒排膿，善透肌肉。

（七）鯽魚灰解毒散堅，醬汁引入蟲口。

（八）冢中石灰專散火毒。

（九）桑灰泄風去熱。

（十）烏羊角灰消堅解毒，相和傅之，尤效。

（十一）丹砂、礬石、雌、雄二黃解毒。

（十二）大黃、黃連滌熱，(竹閒)茹去惡肉敗瘡，莽草治大風壅腫結氣。

Yǎn Yì (Expanded Meaning)

(1) Rooster excrement causes qì to move down and out, and kills worms. By means of the pickling liquid and vinegar, it is drawn in to enter the mouth of the worms.

(2) *Yuánhuā* resolves toxin and kills worms. By means of the lard, it is drawn in to enter the mouth of the worms.

(3) *Tínglì* breaks hardenings, disinhibits water, and kills worms. It is no different than *yuánhuā*.

(4) *Wǔjīng* treats heat toxin and wind swelling.

(5) *Yěgé* treats malign wind and water swelling and kills worms. It is a case of using poison to attack poison.

(6) *Qiūyè* pulls out toxicity and drains pus. It is excellent at outthrusting them from the skin and flesh.

(7) Ashed *jìyú* resolves toxin and dissipates hardenings. By means of the pickling liquid, it is drawn into the worms' mouth.

(8) Lime from inside a tomb specifically dissipates fire toxin.

(9) *Sānggén* ash discharges wind and gets rid of heat.

(10) The ashes of a black sheep or goat horn disperse hardenings and resolves toxins. Combined [with the *sānggén* ashes] and spread on [the sore], they are particularly effective.

(11) *Dānshā, fánshí, cíhuáng,* and *xiónghuáng* resolve toxin.

(12) *Dàhuáng* and *huánglián* flush out heat, *lǜrú* gets rid of malign flesh and vanquished sores, and *mǎngcǎo* treats great wind congestion swelling and bound qì.

（十三）熬豉為末，以除惡毒異氣。

（十四）醋和油煎，專滋風燥。

（十五）皂莢專解風毒。

（十六）胡粉燥濕，乳酥潤燥，燥潤兼濟，專主
月蝕耳瘡剝裂。

（十七）蚓泥、豬膏，清熱解毒。

（十八）灶土、髮灰，收濕散血。

（十九）交道土取其流動，灶下土取其溫暖以治
爛瘡，取其收濕。

（二十）艾葉傅瘡久不斂。

（二十一）牛屎灰傅久瘡滅瘢。

（二十二）竹葉灰和雞子白收濕解毒。

（二十三）髮灰、豬脂，散血潤燥。

（二十四）臭酥、胡粉，潤燥燥濕。

（二十五）麻子潤燥。

(13) Toasted *dòuchǐ* that is pulverized is used to eliminate the malignity, toxicity, and strange qì.

(14) Simmering vinegar and oil specifically moistens wind dryness.

(15) *Zàojiá* specifically resolves wind toxin.

(16) *Húfěn* dries dampness, and butter moistens dryness. Providing relief by simultaneously drying and moistening is specifically indicated for lunar erosion ear sores with peeling and cracking.

(17) Earthworm excrement and lard clear heat and resolve toxin.

(18) Oven earth and ashed hair astringe dampness and disperse blood.

(19) Dirt from a crossroads takes advantage of the activity and flow [in this location], while dirt from underneath the stove takes advantage of its warming and heating power. By means of these, they treat putrefying sores, using their ability to astringe dampness.

(20) *Àiyè* is spread on sores that do not shrink back for a long time.

(21) Applying ashes from cow manure to chronic sores makes scars disappear.

(22) *Zhúyè* ashes mixed with egg white astringes dampness and resolves toxin.

(23) Ashed hair and lard dissipate blood and moisten dryness.

(24) Rancid butter and *húfěn* moisten dryness and dry dampness.

(25) *Mázǐ* moistens dryness.

（二十六）　犬膽殺蟲，犬性熱而膽化熱也。

（二十七）　枸杞清熱散濕。

（二十八）　青核桃皮搗和醋傳去面上濕癬皯皰。

（二十九）　馬尿、牛津、犬屎灰，皆能殺蟲療癬。

（三十）　又取馬尿洗和赤疵，犬屎傳兒身赤黑疵，專取穢以攻血漬也。

（三十一）　針刀抉目疣，膿潰根自落，勝於傳貼也。

(26) The reason why dog bile kills worms is that the inherent [medicinal] quality of dog is hot, and yet the bile transforms heat.

(27) Gǒuqǐ clears heat and dissipates dampness.

(28) Applying green walnut skin that is pounded and mixed with vinegar gets rid of damp ringworm and pimples in the face.

(29) Horse urine, cow saliva, and ashes from dog feces are all able to kill worms and cure ringworm.

(30) Again, using horse urine to wash red blemishes and using dog feces to spread on the red and black blemishes all over a child's body are examples of specifically using filth to attack blood macerations.

(31) Cutting open warts with a needle or knife to cause the pus to burst out and the roots to drop spontaneously is superior to applying plasters.

CHAPTER NINE: MISCELLANEOUS DISEASES OF SMALL CHILDREN

小兒雜病第九

(121 formulas, 13 moxibustion methods)

治小兒臍中生瘡方。

桑汁敷乳上，使兒飲之。

又方
飲羖羊乳及血。

IX.1 Formulas for Treating the Navel

IX.1.a Formulas for Sores in the Navel

Indication
A formula for small children, to treat the formation of sores inside the navel.

Ingredients and Preparation
Apply *sāngyè* juice[1] to the [mother's] breast and then have the child nurse from there.

Another Formula
Drink the milk and blood from a black ewe.[2]

---

1 From similar versions of this formula in other texts, it is clear that this does not refer to juice gained by expressing the berries, as a modern reader might think, but to the juice gained by pounding fresh mulberry leaves into a pulp.

2 According to the *Shuōwén Jiězì*, "female black sheep are called 羖 *gǔ*" (夏羊牡曰羖).

治小兒風臍，遂作惡瘡，歷年不瘥方。

（一）取東壁上土敷之，大佳。

（二）若汁不止，燒蒼耳子粉之。

又方

乾蠐螬蟲末粉之，不過三四度瘥。

Commentary IX.1.b ◆ Sabine Wilms

風臍 *fēng qí*: I have left this term in its literal translation here because I am uncertain of its specific clinical meaning. Unfortunately, the compound is not found in contemporaneous medical texts like the *Zhū Bìng Yuán Hòu Lùn*. Given the context in this chapter, however, we must not confuse it with the much more common expression 臍風 *qí fēng* "umbilical wind"! "Umbilical wind" is a technical term referring to a critical pediatric condition roughly equivalent to neonatal tetanus, contracted due to improper cutting of the umbilical cord and care of the umbilicus immediately after birth. See the discussion of this condition in Chapter Two of Volume Five ("Emergence of the Newborn from the Abdomen"), translated and commented on in Venerating the Root, Part One, pp. 56-57. By contrast, the term *fēng qí* ("wind navel") here must describe a chronic skin condition of oozing sores in the navel that is for some unknown reason associated with wind, most likely as an etiological agent. This is confirmed by the use of the term in other medical texts, such as the *Qí Xiào Liáng Fāng* 《奇效良方》 ("Excellent Formulas with Wondrous Efficacy," completed in 1449), which includes a formula for a decoction to treat "wind umbilicus and water umbilicus with swelling and festering in small children" (小兒風臍水臍，腫爛), to be applied to the umbilicus three to four times a day.

IX.1.b Formulas for "Wind Navel"

Indication
A formula for small children, to treat "wind navel," which subsequently causes malign sores and persists for years without healing.

Ingredients and Preparation
(1) Take dirt from the top of the eastern wall[3] and spread it on [the navel]. This is most excellent.

(2) If the liquid[4] does not stop, toast *cāngěrzǐ* and sprinkle this on [the sores].

Another Formula
Process dried *qícǎo* bugs into a powder and sprinkle it on [the sores]. After no more than three or four treatments, [the sores] will have healed.

---

3   This denotes a substance with great yáng characteristics since the eastern wall receives the influence of the morning sun.

4   Most likely, this refers to the liquid oozing from the sores in the navel.

治小兒臍不合方。

大車轄脂燒灰，日一敷之。

又方
燒蜂房灰末，敷之。

治小兒臍中生瘡方

燒甀帶灰，和膏敷之。

IX.1.c Formulas for Failure of the Navel to Close

Indication
A formula to treat small children with a navel that will not close.

Ingredients and Preparation
Char the grease from the linchpin of a large cart into ashes and spread this [on the navel] once a day.

Another Formula
Char a beehive into ashes and spread this [on the navel].

IX.1.d Formula for Sores in the Navel

Indication
A formula for small children, to treat the formation of sores inside the navel.

Ingredients and Preparation
Char the band around a steaming pot[5] into ashes, mix it with salve, and apply it.

---

5 甑帶 *zèng dài*: Literally "band of a steaming pot." While historical steaming implements could be constructed from wood or clay or even bronze, the clay radical in the character 甑 *zèng* suggests that it most likely derived originally from a clay vessel. It originally referred to a two-part container that was suspended on a metal tripod, with holes in the bottom of the top part to allow the steam from below to enter and cook the food that had been placed in the upper portion. The "band" of the steamer was presumably a cord that was wrapped around the vessel to assist in lifting it onto and off of its base. According to the *Zhènglèi Běncǎo*, the ashes from the band of a steaming vessel are a medicinal ingredient for abdominal Distension and pain and for rectal prolapse. Simmered in liquid and administered orally, this substance is indicated for stomach reflux; urinary incontinence, stoppage and strangury; malignity strike and corpse influx; and metal wounds. A commentary quoted there states that the "band" around the steamer is made from cattail in Jīngnán, and that you should choose one that has been in use for a long time since it is imbued with steam and is therefore particularly effective at dissipating and unblocking qì.

治小兒臍赤腫方。

杏仁	半兩
豬頰車髓	十八銖

上二味，先研杏仁如脂，和髓敷臍中腫上。

白石脂散

治小兒臍汁不止，兼赤腫方。

以白石脂細研，熬令微暖，以粉臍瘡，日三四度。

IX.1.e Formula for a Red and Swollen Navel

Indication

A formula for small children, to treat redness and swelling of the navel.

Ingredients

xìngrén	0.5 *liǎng*
marrow from a pig's lower jaw	18 *zhū*

Preparation

Of the two ingredients above, first grind the *xìngrén* into a paste, then combine it with the marrow and apply it to the swelling inside the navel.

IX.1.f Báishízhī Sǎn (Kaolin Powder)

Indication

A formula for small children, to treat incessant oozing from the navel that is accompanied by redness and swelling.

Ingredients and Preparation

Finely grind *báishízhī* and heat it up until slightly warm. Sprinkle this on the sores in the navel, three to four times a day.

衍義

（一）桑汁解風熱。

（二）羖羊乳滋血燥。

（三）東壁土燥濕。

（四）蒼耳灰去風濕斂汗。

（五）蟛蜞破血，乾末粉身，奪血止汗。

（六）車脂灰通血脈滋燥。

（七）蜂房灰攻毒去風。

（八）甑帶灰通津收濕。

（九）杏仁、豬髓，解毒滋燥。

（十）白石脂固脫杜風。

（十一）各詳見證取用。

Formulas for Treating the Navel, *Yǎn Yì* (Expanded Meaning)

(1) *Sāngyè* juice resolves wind heat.

(2) Milk from a black ewe irrigates blood dryness.

(3) Dirt from an east-facing wall dries dampness.

(4) *Cāngěr* [charred into] ashes gets rid of wind-damp and constrains sweating.

(5) *Qícǎo* breaks up blood and, when dried, pulverized, and sprinkled on the body, wrests away the blood and stops sweating.

(6) Cart grease [charred into] ashes opens up the flow of blood in the vessels and irrigates dryness.

(7) A beehive [charred into] ashes attacks toxin and gets rid of wind.

(8) Steaming pot bands [charred into] ashes opens up the flow of the liquids and astringes dampness.

(9) *Xìngrén* and pig marrow resolve toxins and irrigate dryness.

(10) *Báishízhī* secures desertion and shuts out wind.

(11) In each case, carefully look at the symptoms and then select the [correct] application.

治小兒鵝口不能飲乳方。

鵝屎汁瀝兒口中。

又方

黍米汁塗之。

又方

（一）取小兒父母亂髮，淨洗，纏桃枝沾取井花
水。

（二）東向向日以髮拭口中白乳。

（三）以置水中七過，瀝洗，三朝作之。

Commentary IX.2 ✒ Sabine Wilms

鵝口 *é kǒu*: Literally translated, this term means "goose mouth." I
have chosen the biomedical identification because "thrush" has a
large enough and closely overlapping range of meaning to serve
as an equivalent. According to the Merriam-Webster Collegiate
Dictionary, thrush is defined as "a disease that is caused by a
fungus (Candida albicans), occurs especially in infants and children, and is marked by white patches in the oral cavity." According to the pertinent entry in the pediatric section of the *Zhū Bìng
Yuán Hòu Lùn*, "When small children are first born, white particles
rise up in the mouth, which then cause sores to form on the top
of the tongue. Since they look like the inside of a goose's mouth,
everybody calls [this condition] 'goose mouth.' This [condition] is
caused by the fetus receiving an exuberance of grain qì in utero,
as a result of which the qì fumes up from the heart and spleen and
erupts in the mouth."

IX.2 Formulas for Mouth Sores

IX.2.a Thrush

Indication
A formula to treat thrush in small children, which is preventing them from nursing.

Ingredients and Preparation
Drip liquid goose droppings into the child's mouth.

Another Formula
Coat [the child's mouth] with broomcorn millet juice.[6]

Another Formula
1) Take *luànfà* from the child's parents, wash it clean, and wind it around a peach wood branch. Dip this in well flower water. [7]

2) [Make the patient] face east and the [early morning] sun. With the hair, wipe down the white milk[-like patches] inside the [patient's] mouth.

3) Place [the hair] in the water seven times and then drizzle [the water into the mouth] and wash out [the mouth]. Do this for three mornings.

---

6 Internally, broomcorn millet (*shǔmǐ*) is administered as a decoction, a gruel, or, as in the present formula, as simply the liquid gained from rinsing it, which is more commonly referred to as 泔汁 *gān zhī*.

7 井花水 *jǐng huā shuǐ*: This is a technical term that refers to the first water drawn from a well in the morning.

Commentary IX.2 ⋅ Julian Scott

"Exuberance of grain": In modern society it would be excessive sugar intake, as well as too much carbohydrate.

治小兒心熱，口為生瘡，重舌鵝口方。

（一）柘根銼五升，無根弓材亦佳。

（二）以水五升，煮取二升，去滓更煎，取五合。

（三）細細敷之，數數為之良。

治口瘡白漫漫方。

取桑汁，先以父髮拭口，以桑汁塗之。

IX.2.b Formula for Heart Heat

Indication

A formula for small children, to treat "heart heat" with the formation of sores in the mouth, Double Tongue,[8] and thrush.

Ingredients and Preparation

(1) Finely shave 5 *shēng* of *zhègēn*.[9] If you do not have any of this root, wood used for making bows is also excellent.

(2) Decoct [the shavings] in 5 *shēng* of water until reduced to 2 *shēng*. Remove the dregs and simmer it again until reduced to 5 *gě*.

(3) Applying it very delicately in numerous repetitions is best.

IX.2.c Formula for Mouth Sores with White Inundation

Indication

A formula to treat mouth sores with white inundation.

Ingredients and Preparation

Take *sāngyè* juice. First wipe out the mouth with hair from [the patient's] father, then daub on the *sāngyè* juice.

---

8 See chapter IX.3.a below for more information on "Double Tongue."

9 柘根 *zhè gēn*: This refers to the root of *zhèmù*, i.e., Cudrania or silkworm thorn.

衍義

（一）鵝屎汁截風解毒。

（二）黍米汁清胃化熱。

（三）淨髮拭口去熱毒。

（四）柘根除腎經風熱。

（五）桑汁清肺熱，口白則胎毒上迫於肺也。

Formulas for Mouth Sores *Yǎn Yì* (Expanded Meaning)

(1) The liquid from goose droppings interrupts wind and resolves toxin.

(2) Cornbroom millet juice clears the stomach and transforms heat.

(3) Wiping out the mouth with clean hair gets rid of heat toxin.

(4) *Zhègēn* eliminates wind heat from the kidney channel.

(5) *Sāngyè* juice clears lung heat. The whiteness in the mouth means that fetal toxin has moved up to distress the lung.

治重舌舌強，不能放唾方。

鹿角末如大豆許，安舌下，日三四度。
亦治小兒不能乳。

又方

取蛇蛻燒末，以雞毛蘸醇醋點藥，掠舌下愈。

Commentary IX.3 ぺ Sabine Wilms

重舌 *chóng shé*: The character 重 can be read either as *zhòng*, in which case it means "heavy," or as *chóng*, in which case it means "double." At first glance, the translation of this symptom as "heavy tongue" might seem more likely since it is easier for us to think of a "heavy" tongue as an equivalent to the English "tongue-tied" than the exotic-sounding notion of a literal "double tongue." Nevertheless, my reading of 重 here as *chóng* is based on the explanation of this disease in the *Zhū Bìng Yuán Hòu Lùn*. According to the pertinent entry in volume 48, "The pediatric condition of Double Tongue is caused by heat in the heart and spleen. The heart manifests its symptoms in the tongue and governs the blood. The network vessels of the spleen, furthermore, emerge below the tongue. Heart fire and spleen earth, these two viscera stand in a mother-child relationship. The presence of heat [in either of them] results in exuberance of both qì and blood. Its manifestation is an attachment below the tongue, near the root of the tongue, forming a shape like a tongue but shorter. Therefore it is called 'double tongue.'"

IX.3 Formulas for Double Tongue

IX.3.a Unnamed Formula

Indication

A formula to treat Double Tongue rigidity[10] of the tongue, and inability to release[11] saliva.

Ingredients and Preparation

Pulverize an amount of *lùjiǎo* roughly equivalent to a soybean and place it under [the patient's] tongue, three to four times a day.

This [formula] is also a treatment for small children being unable to nurse.

Another Formula

Take *shétuìpí* and char and pulverize it. With a chicken feather dipped in unadulterated vinegar, dab the medicine on. Brushing the [area] beneath the tongue [causes] recovery.

---

10 Editorial comment: The *Sūn Zhēnrén* edition has 腫 *zhǒng* ("swelling") here instead of 強 *qiáng* ("rigidity").

11 Editorial comment: A number of other editions, including the *Yǎn Yì*, have 收 *shōu* "gather in/astringe" here instead of 放 *fàng* ("release").

Commentary IX.3 ❧ Julian Scott

I presume this refers to the fold of skin that can hold the tongue to the floor of the mouth, causing a condition referred to as "tongue-tied" in common English or as ankyloglossia as the technical term. In the past, the family doctor used to cut it with scissors, but there are risks: One in a thousand people (babies and adults) have an artery that goes there, and there is a real risk of bleeding to death. I knew a singer who had his cut when he was in his later twenties, and he very nearly died of anaemia.

治小兒重舌方。

田中蜂房燒灰，酒和，塗喉下愈。

又方
衣魚塗舌上。

又方
竈月下黃土末，苦酒和塗舌上。

IX.3.b Formulas for Double Tongue

Unnamed Formula
Indication
A formula for small children, to treat double tongue.

Ingredients and Preparation
Char a beehive from the middle of a field into ashes and mix it with liquor. Applying it below the throat[12] causes recovery.

Another Formula
Apply silverfish to the top of the tongue.

Another Formula
Take yellow dirt from inside the stove, pulverize it, mix it with bitter liquor, and apply it to the top of the tongue.

---

12   While it is possible that "throat" could be a textual corruption and should be replaced with "tongue" here, since the formula concerns the treatment of the region below the tongue, that is unlikely, given that the various editions of the *Qiān Jīn Fāng* all repeat this exact wording.

又方

三家屠肉，切令如指大，摩舌上，兒立能啼。

又方

赤小豆末，醋和塗舌上。

又方

燒簸箕灰敷舌上。

又方

黃柏以竹瀝漬，取細細點舌上，良。

Another Formula

Have three households slaughter meat[13] and cut it into finger-sized pieces. Rub the top of the [child's] tongue with this, and the child will immediately be able to wail.

Another Formula

Pulverize *chìxiǎodòu* and mix it with vinegar. Spread this on the top of the tongue.

Another Formula

Char a winnowing basket into ashes and spread this on the top of the tongue.[14]

Another Formula

Soak *huángbò* in *zhúlì*. Take this and drip it very delicately on the top of the tongue. It is excellent.

---

13 The exact meaning of this instruction is unclear to me. It could mean that this treatment requires three different batches of meat, from three different households who each slaughtered their meat independently, or that three households collaborated in a sort of communal slaughtering, and that you merely need a single piece of meat, roughly finger-sized, which you use to rub the top of the patient's tongue. The latter explanation seems a bit more likely to me, given that it would be difficult to fit more than a single piece of meat in a small child's mouth to perform this treatment.

14 Editorial comment: This formula is missing in many editions, including the *Yǎn Yì*.

重舌，灸行間隨年壯，穴在足大趾歧中。

又
灸兩足外踝上三壯。

IX.4 Moxibustion Treatments for Double Tongue

Unnamed Method

For Double Tongue, burn moxa on Xíngjiān,[15] the number of cones being identical to the [patient's] age. The point is located in the center of the divergence of the big toe.

Another [Method]

Burn three cones of moxa [each] on top of the lateral ankle on both feet.[16]

---

15 行間 xíng jiān: "Moving Between," now identified with LV-2.

16 This location is identical with the point Wàihuáijiān, used in modern TCM primarily in bleeding and moxa treatments, to address tooth problems, strangury, beriberi, localized cramping, inflammation of the tonsils, and Double Tongue. According to Julian Scott, the tip of the external malleolus treats the jaw and tongue. In vol. 21 of the *Qiān Jīn Fāng*, the point is used to treat sudden strangury.

治小兒舌上瘡方。

蜂房燒灰、屋間塵各等分，和勻敷之。

又方
桑白汁塗乳，與兒飲之。

又方
羊蹄骨中生髓，和胡粉敷之。

治舌腫強滿方。

滿口含糖醋良。

又方
飲羖羊乳即瘥。

IX.5 Other Tongue Problems

IX.5.a Formulas for Sores on the Tongue

Unnamed Formula
Indication
A formula for small children, to treat sores on top of the tongue.

Ingredients and Preparation
Take equal amounts of beehive charred into ashes and dust from inside the house. Mix them until blended evenly and spread on [the sores].

Another Formula
Spread *sāngbái* juice[17] on the [mother's] breast and have the child nurse from there.

Another Formula
Take the marrow from the middle of a goat or sheep's hoof, mix it with *húfěn*, and spread it on [the sores].

IX.5.b Formulas for Swollen Tongue

Unnamed Formula
Indication
A formula to treat swelling, rigidity, and fullness of the tongue.

Ingredients and Preparation
Fill the mouth with malt sugar and vinegar and hold it there. This is excellent.

Another Formula
Drinking milk from a black ewe causes immediate recovery.

---

17 This term is identical with *sāngyè* juice. See note 1 on page 335 above.

衍義

（一）鹿角治惡血散熱腫。

（二）蛇蛻截風毒。

（三）蜂房投驚痰。

（四）衣魚散風癎。

（五）灶土斂虛陽。

（六）赤小豆解熱毒。

（七）竹瀝漬黃柏，解胎熱，去痰涎。

（八）蜂房、桑汁，並解熱毒。

（九）羊蹄髓和胡粉，鎮攝肺胃風熱。

（十）糖醋斂肝脾之火。

（十一）羖羊乳潤燥舒筋，關一切不正之氣。

Treatments for Tongue Problems *Yăn Yì* (Expanded Meaning)

(1) *Lùjiăo* treats malign blood and dissipates heat swelling.

(2) *Shétuì* interrupts wind toxin.

(3) Beehive throws out fright phlegm.

(4) Silverfish dissipate wind seizures.

(5) Yellow dirt from inside the stove restrains vacuous yáng.

(6) *Chìxiăodòu* resolves heat toxin.

(7) *Huángbò* soaked in *zhúlì* resolves fetal heat and gets rid of phlegm-drool.

(8) Beehive and *sāngyè* juice both resolve heat toxin.

(9) The combination of marrow from a goat or sheep's hoof and *húfěn* quells and captures wind and heat in the lung and stomach.

(10) Malt sugar and vinegar restrain fire in the liver and spleen.

(11) Milk from a black ewe moistens dryness and soothes the sinews, while also repelling all qì that is not right.

治小兒口瘡不得吮乳方。

大青	十八銖
黃連	十二銖

（一）上二味，咬咀，以水三升，煮取一升二
合。

（二）一服一合，日再夜一。

又方

臘月豬脂	一斤
蜜	二斤
甘草	如指大三寸

上三味，合煎相得，含如棗大，稍稍咽之，日
三。

IX.6 Treatments for Mouth Problems

IX.6.a Formulas for Mouth Sores

Unnamed Formula
Indication
A formula for small children, to treat mouth sores that are preventing them from sucking on the breast.

Ingredients

dàqīng	18 *zhū*
huánglián	12 *zhū*

Preparation
(1) Pound the two ingredients above and decoct in 3 *shēng* of water until reduced to 1 *shēng* and 2 *gě*.

(2) A single dose is 1 *gě*, taken twice during the day and once at night.

Another Formula
Ingredients

làyuèzhūzhī	1 *jīn*
honey	2 *jīn*
gāncǎo	a finger-sized piece, 3 *cùn* long

Preparation
Combine the three ingredients above and simmer until everything is mixed well. [Have the patient] hold a piece about the size of a jujube in the mouth and little by little swallow it down. [Repeat this treatment] three times a day.

又方

礜石如雞子大，置醋中，塗兒足下二七遍愈。

治小兒燕口，兩吻生瘡方。

燒髮灰和豬脂敷之。

Commentary IX.6.b ✦ Sabine Wilms

This is a literal translation of the Chinese term 燕口 *yàn kǒu*, which is described as follows in vol. 30 of the *Zhū Bìng Yuán Hòu Lùn*: "Foot Tàiyīn is the Spleen Channel and its qì penetrates to the mouth. Foot Yángmíng is the Stomach Channel, and Hand Yángmíng is the Large Intestine Channel. These two channels both run right along the mouth. Vacuity in these organs allows the evils of wind and dampness to take advantage of [the situation]. Their qì erupts in the vessels and struggles with the fluids, as a result of which sores form. They are permanently damp, putrefying, and purulent. Commonly called 'fat sores,' they are also called 'swallow mouth sores.'" According to the entry on "Swallow Mouth" in the pediatric volume of the *Zhū Bìng Yuán Hòu Lùn* (volume 50), "The condition is caused by heat intruding into the spleen and stomach. The heat qì fumes up and erupts in the mouth, causing the formation of sores on both lips. The sores are white, resembling the lips of a swallow, which is the reason why the condition is named Swallow Mouth sores."

Another Formula

Place a piece of *fánshí* about the size of a chicken egg in vinegar. Apply this to the bottom of the child's feet. After two times seven rounds [of treatment, the patient] will recover.

IX.6.b Formula for Swallow Mouth

Indication

A formula for small children, to treat Swallow Mouth with sores forming on both lips.

Ingredients and Preparation

Char hair into ashes and combine with lard. Spread it on [the sores].

Commentary IX.6 ✤ Julian Scott

The large number of formulas for mouth problems is undoubtedly related to the fact that the baby will not suckle properly if there is a problem in the mouth. Not eating enough in a cold climate means almost certain death for a baby. In the West we have central heating, and there is always the last resort of feeding via a nasal tube.

治小兒口下黃肌瘡方。

（一）取羖羊髭燒灰，和臘月豬脂敷之。
（二）角亦可用。

治口旁惡瘡方。

亂髮灰
故絮灰
黃連
乾薑

上四味，等分，為散，以粉瘡上，不過三遍。

IX.6.c Formula for Yellow Flesh and Sores on the Bottom of the Mouth

Indication

A formula for small children, to treat yellow flesh and sores on the bottom of the mouth.[18]

Ingredients and Preparation

(1) Take the whiskers from a black ewe and char them into ashes. Combine with *làyuèzhūzhī* and spread it on [the sores and yellow flesh].

(2) You can also use the horn [from a black ewe].

IX.6.d Formula for Malign Sores

Indication

A formula to treat malign sores on the sides of the mouth.

Ingredients

luànfà, ashed
old silk wadding, ashed
huánglián
gānjiāng

Preparation

Take equal amounts of the four ingredients above and make a powder. Sprinkle this on the sores. Do not exceed three applications.

---

18 口下 *kǒu xià*: Literally "below the mouth." Given the context of this formula in a chapter on problems of the mouth and its position within the chapter in a section on sores inside the mouth, I have chosen to translate 下 in the sense of "lower part," and therefore "bottom" in the line above, instead of "underneath."

治口噤，赤者心噤，白者肺噤方。

雞屎白棗大，綿裹，以水一合，煮二沸，分再
服。

治小兒口噤方。

| 鹿角粉 |
| 大豆末 |

上二味，等分，和乳塗乳上，飲兒。

IX.6.e Formula for Clenched Jaw

Indication
A formula to treat clenched jaw. When it is red, it means heart clenching, and when it is white, lung clenching.

Ingredients and Preparation
Take an amount of chicken manure roughly the size of a jujube, wrap it in silk floss, and decoct it in 1 *gě* of water, bringing it to a boil twice. Divide and give in two doses.

IX.6.f More Formulas for Clenched Jaw

Unnamed Formula
Indication
A formula for small children, to treat clenched jaw.

Ingredients

lùjiǎo, powdered
dàdòu, pulverized

Preparation
Take equal amounts of the two ingredients above, mix with [breast] milk, and spread on the breast. Have the child nurse from there.

又方

驢乳	各一升
豬乳	

上二味，合煎，得一升五合，服如杏仁許，三四
服瘥。

雀屎丸

主小兒卒中風，口噤，不下一物方。

（一）雀屎如麻子，丸之，飲下即愈，大良。

（二）雞屎白亦佳。

Another formula

Ingredients[19]

donkey milk	1 *shēng* each
pig milk	

Preparation

Simmer the two ingredients above together until reduced to 1 *shēng* and 5 *gě*. Give an amount about the size of an apricot pit per dose. Three or four doses will cure [the condition].

IX.6.g Quèshǐ Wán (Sparrow Droppings Pill)

Indication

A formula indicated for small children, to treat sudden wind strike with clenched jaw and failure to get [even] a single substance down.[20]

Ingredients and Preparation

(1) Take an amount of sparrow droppings roughly the size of a hemp seed and form it into a pill. Getting it down in liquid leads to immediate recovery. This is very excellent.

(2) The white in chicken droppings is also excellent.

---

19   Several other editions, including the *Yǎn Yì*, have 二升 *èr shēng* ("two *shēng*") instead, in which case you would simply boil down the milk into a much more concentrated preparation.

20   In other words, the patient is so ill that it is impossible to make her or him ingest anything at all. This description would make it quite difficult, however, to get the patient to take the medicine. One possible, but in my opinion highly unlikely, explanation could be to read 下 *xià* in the sense of "moving [a substance] down and out of the body," or in other words, eliminating it through urination or defecation. A more likely interpretation is that the patient is unable to get anything down on his or her own, to actively ingest anything, but that it is still possible to force a medicine down the patient's throat.

治小兒口中涎出方。

以白羊屎納口中。

又方
以東行牛口中沫，塗口中及頤上。

又方
桑白汁塗之瘥。

IX.6.h Formulas for Drooling

Unnamed Formula
Indication
A formula for small children, to treat drooling from inside the mouth.

Ingredients and Preparation
Take excrement from a white sheep or goat and put it inside the [patient's] mouth.

Another Formula
Take saliva from inside the mouth of an ox that is walking towards the east. Spread this on the inside of [the patient's] mouth and on the lower jaws.

Another Formula
Spreading *sāngbáizhǐ* [on the inside of the mouth?] will cause recovery.

衍義

（一）大青、黃連治肝脾實火。

（二）甘蜜、豬脂散脾胃虛火。

（三）醋、礬、雞清收斂濕熱。

（四）髮灰解毒散惡血。

（五）羖羊須散血收濕。

（六）髮絮灰、姜、連末散血導火。

（七）雞屎白下氣袪風。

（八）鹿角、豆末散血解毒。

（九）驢豬乳潤燥化風熱。

（十）雀屎闢風毒開噤。

（十一）羊矢去火毒化風熱。

（十二）牛涎解脾胃蘊熱。

（十三）又桑白汁解肺胃風熱，分主手足太陰風燥。

Treatments for Mouth Problems *Yǎn Yì* (Expanded Meaning)

(1) *Dàqīng* and *huánglián* treat repletion fire in the liver and spleen.

(2) Honey and lard dissipate vacuity fire in the spleen and stomach.

(3) Vinegar, *fánshí*, and chicken clear, gather in, and restrain damp-heat.

(4) Hair [charred into] ashes resolves toxin and dissipates malign blood.

(5) Whiskers from a black ewe dissipate blood and astringe dampness.

(6) The powder made from ashed *luànfà* and silk wadding, *gānjiāng*, and *huánglián* dissipates blood and abducts fire.

(7) The white in chicken droppings brings down qì and dispels wind.

(8) Pulverized *lùjiǎo* and *dàdòu* dissipate blood and resolve toxin.

(9) Donkey milk and pig milk irrigate dryness and transform wind heat.

(10) Sparrow droppings repel wind toxin and open up clenching.

(11) Goat or sheep excrement gets rid of fire toxin and transforms wind heat.

(12) Ox saliva resolves heat brewing in the spleen and stomach.

(13) And lastly, *sāngbáizhǐ* resolves wind heat in the lung and stomach. It separately rules wind dryness in Hand and Foot Tàiyīn.

治小兒卒毒腫著喉頸，壯熱妨乳方。

升麻	
射乾	各一兩
大黃	

（一）上三味，咬咀，以水一升五合，煮取八合。

（二）一歲兒分五服，以滓薄腫上，冷更暖以薄，大兒以意加之。

IX.7 Treatments for Throat Conditions

IX.7.a Formula for Sudden Toxin Swelling

Indication

A formula for small children, to treat sudden toxin swelling affecting the throat and neck, with vigorous heat effusion and an obstruction to [the patient's ability to] nurse.

Ingredients

shēngmá	
shègān	1 *liǎng* each
dàhuáng	

Preparation

(1) Pound the three ingredients above and simmer in 1 *shēng* and 5 *gě* of water until reduced to 8 *gě*.

(2) For a child of one *suì*, divide into five doses.[21] Take [some of] the dregs and spread them thinly on the swelling. When they have cooled off, replace them with warm [dregs to apply] another thin layer. For an older child, increase [the dosage] at your discretion.

---

21 I have left the translation literally, in spite of the fact that there is an ambiguity on whether these instructions imply that the patient should ingest the medicine in five doses as well as receiving the external treatment or whether the entire treatment consists of the external applications of the sediment from the decoction. That seems unlikely, though, given that the decoction is divided into five doses. Also, the character 服 *fú* means not only "dose" but also "to ingest," and can be used in such a way as to refer to "ingesting in [x number of] doses." It is most likely that the line here is intended in this way and should therefore be read as "For a child of one to four *suì*, have them ingest it in five doses."

升麻湯

治小兒喉痛，若毒氣盛，便咽塞，並主大人咽喉不利方。

升麻	
生薑	各二兩
射乾	
橘皮	一兩

上四味，咬咀，以水六升，煮取二升，去滓，分三服。

治小兒喉痹腫方。

魚膽二七枚，以和竈底土塗之，瘥止。

IX.7.b Shēngmá Tāng (Cimicifuga Decoction)

Indication

A formula for small children, to treat pain in the throat, as if from an exuberance of toxic qì, followed immediately by throat congestion. It also rules inhibition in the throat in adults.

Ingredients

shēngmá	
shēngjiāng	2 *liǎng* each
shègān	
júpí	1 *liǎng*

Preparation

Pound the four ingredients above and simmer in 6 *shēng* of water until reduced to 2 *shēng*. Remove the dregs and divide into three doses.

IX.7.c Formula for Throat Impediment with Swelling

Indication

A formula for small children, to treat throat *bì* impediment and swelling.

Ingredients and Preparation

Take two times seven fish gallbladders and mix with earth from the bottom of a stove.[22] Spreading it on [the throat] results in recovery and in stopping [the problem].

---

22 竈底土 *zào dǐ tǔ*: This is a common medicinal ingredient, usually referred to as *zàozhōnghuángtǔ* or, in more modern texts, as 伏龍肝 *fú lóng gān*.

治小兒喉痹方。

桂心	各半兩
杏仁	

上二味，末之，以綿裹如棗大，含咽汁。

IX.7.d Formula for Throat Impediment

Indication

A formula to treat throat *bì* impediment in small children.

Ingredients

guìxīn	0.5 *liǎng* each
xìngrén	

Preparation

Pulverize the two ingredients above and wrap an amount about as big as a jujube in silk floss. [Have the patient] hold it in the mouth and swallow the juice.

衍義

（一）升麻上引，大黃下泄，射乾專散咽喉結氣，取其先升後降也。

（二）升麻引射乾上行散結。

（三）姜、橘開提痰氣。

（四）鯖魚膽苦寒，專散肝膽之火。

（五）竈土專化脾胃之熱。

（六）桂心導龍火。

（七）杏仁下結氣。

（八）從治之法也。

Treatments for Throat Conditions *Yǎn Yì* (Expanded Meaning)

(1) *Shēngmá* draws upward while *dàhuáng* drains downward. *Shègān* specifically dissipates bound qì in the throat. [This formula] applies [the treatment method] of first upbearing and then downbearing.

(2) *Shēngmá* draws *shègān* upward to dissipate binds.

(3) *Shēngjiāng* and *júpí* open up and lift phlegm qì.

(4) Carp gallbladders[23] are bitter and cold and specifically dissipate fire from the liver and gallbladder.

(5) Stove earth specifically transforms heat in the spleen and stomach.

(6) *Guìxīn* abducts dragon fire.[24]

(7) *Xìngrén* moves down bound qì.

(8) This is the method of "co-acting treatment."[25]

---

23 I interpret the character 鯖 *qīng* in the compound 鯖魚 *qīng yú* here as a scribal error for 青魚 *qīng yú* (Mylopharyngodonis Caro, "Black Carp"), because the bile of that fish species is commonly used in Chinese medicine as a medicinal ingredient, while the former (Scomber scombrus, "Atlantic mackerel") is not traditionally used for that purpose.

24 According to the section on fire in the *Běncǎo Gāngmù*, fire can be differentiated as yīn fire and yáng fire. Regarding yīn fire, "Heaven has two kinds of yīn fire: dragon fire and thunder fire." On the other hand, "dragon fire" is also an alternate name for the lunar mansion more commonly referred to as the "heart mansion" (心宿 *xīn sù*), which is one of the seven constellations in the east, because these in turn are referred to as 蒼龍 *cāng lóng* ("Azure Dragon").

25 This means treating like with like, as in treating heat with heat above

治小兒解顱方。

熬蛇蛻皮，末之，和豬頰車中髓，敷頂上，日三四度。

又方
豬牙頰車髓敷囟上瘥。

IX.8 Treatments for Skull Problems

IX.8.a Formulas for Separated Cranial Bones

Indication
A formula for small children, to treat separated cranial bones.

Ingredients and Preparation
Roast *shétuìpí* and pulverize it. Mix it with the marrow from inside a pig's lower jaw and apply this to the top of the head, three to four times a day.

Another Formula
Applying the marrow from a pig's lower jaw on top of the fontanels will lead to recovery.

Commentary IX.8.a ᴥ Sabine Wilms

解顱 *jiě lú*: I translate this technical term literally as "separated cranial bones" based on the explanation of this condition in the *Zhū Bìng Yuán Hòu Lùn*. It refers quite literally to a failure of the fontanels, the spaces between the cranial bones in an infant's head, to close up as they should, by age 2 in the case of the anterior fontanel and by 18 months in the case of the posterior one. The *Zhū Bìng Yuán Hòu Lùn* defines it as "In appearance, if small children grow older in age when the [fontanels between the] skull [bones] should close up, but they fail to do so, and the seams in the head remain open, this is it. It is caused by a failure to complete the formation of the kidney qì. The kidney rules the bones and marrow, and the brain is the Sea of Marrow. When the formation of kidney qì is incomplete, the marrow and brain are insufficient so they are unable to complete the process of binding together. For this reason, the skull bones remain separated.

半夏熨湯

治小兒腦長，解顱不合，羸瘦色黃，至四五歲不
能行方。

半夏	各一升
生薑	
芎藭	
細辛	三兩
桂心	一尺
烏頭	十枚

（一）上六味，㕮咀，以醇苦酒五升，漬之。晬
　　　時，煮三沸，絞去滓。

（二）以綿一片浸藥中，適寒溫以熨囟上，冷更
　　　溫之，複熨如前。

（三）朝暮各三四熨乃止，二十日愈。

IX.8.b Bànxià Yùn Tāng (Pinellia Hot Compress Decoction)

Indication

A formula for small children, to treat [pathological] growing of the brain[26] and separated cranial bones that are failing to close, with marked emaciation and a yellow complexion and inability to walk all the way to the age of four or five *suì*.

Ingredients

bànxià	
shēngjiāng	1 *shēng* each
xiōngqióng	
xìxīn	3 *liǎng*
guìxīn	1 *chǐ*
wūtóu	10 pieces

Preparation

(1) Pound the six ingredients above and soak in 5 *shēng* of pure bitter liquor. At the time of the first birthday anniversary, simmer it, bringing it to a boil three times, and then wring it out and remove the dregs.

(2) Take a piece of silk floss and soak it in the medicine. Apply this at a comfortable temperature as a compress to the fontanels. When it has cooled off, replace it with a warm one and again apply the compress as before.

(3) Apply three to four compresses every morning and evening and then stop. After twenty days, the patient will be cured.

---

26 腦長 *nǎo zhǎng*: The character 長 can be read as *cháng*, in which case it means "long" or "to lengthen," or as *zhǎng*, in which case it means "to grow," "to increase in size." My best guess is that the expression "growing of the brain" here refers to a pathological expansion of the brain that is preventing the fontanels from closing by putting pressure on the cranial bones from the inside.

生蟹足敷方

治小兒解顱方。

生蟹足	各半兩
白蘞	

上二味，搗末，以乳汁和，敷顱上，立愈。

三物細辛敷方

治小兒解顱方。

細辛	各半兩
桂心	
乾薑	十八銖

（一）上末之，以淳汁和，敷顱上。

（二）乾複敷之，兒面赤即愈。

IX.8.c Shēngxièzú Fū Fāng (Raw Crab Legs Spread-On Formula)

Indication

A formula for small children, to treat separated cranial bones.

Ingredients

shēngxièzú	0.5 *liǎng* each
báiliǎn	

Preparation

Pound the two ingredients above into a powder and combine with breast milk. Spread on the skull, and immediate recovery will ensue.

IX.8.d Sān Wù Xìxīn Fū Fāng (Three-Ingredients Asarum Spread-On Formula)

Indication

A formula for small children, to treat separated cranial bones.

Ingredients

xìxīn	0.5 *liǎng* each
guìxīn	
gānjiāng	18 *zhū*

Preparation

(1) Pulverize the ingredients above and combine with breast milk. Spread on the skull.

(2) When it has dried, repeat the application. When the child's face turns red, this means recovery.

治小兒囟開不合方。

防風	一兩半
柏子	各一兩
白茋	

（一）上三味，末之，以乳和敷囟上。

（二）十日知，二十日即愈，日一。

又方

取豬牙車骨煎取髓，敷囟上愈。

小兒囟陷，灸臍上下各半寸，及鳩尾骨端，又足太陰，各一壯。

Commentary IX.8.d ᴥ Sabine Wilms

Caved-in Fontanels: See the pertinent entry in the *Zhū Bìng Yuán Hòu Lùn* vol. 48, which explains caved-in fontanels as follows: "This is caused by the presence of heat in the intestines, heat qì smoldering in the *zàng* organs, and the heat in the *zàng* organs causing thirst and drawing rheum. When urination is [at the same time] disinhibited and urine is discharged, the blood and qì in the *zàng* and *fǔ* organs becomes vacuous and weak. It is unable to ascend and fill the marrow and brain. As a result, the fontanels cave in."

IX.8.e Formulas for Open Fontanels

Indication

A formula for small children, to treat open fontanels that are failing to close.

Ingredients

fángfēng	1.5 *liǎng*
bǎizǐ	1 *liǎng* each
báijī	

Preparation

(1) Pulverize the three ingredients above and combine with breast milk. Spread on the fontanels.

(2) After ten days, you will notice [an effect], and after twenty days, [the patient] will be cured. [Apply] once a day.

Another Formula

Roast a pig's lower jaw and take the marrow. Spread this on the fontanels. Recovery will ensue.

IX.8.f Moxibustion Method

For caved-in fontanels in small children, burn moxa half a *cùn* above and below the navel, as well as on the very end of the xiphoid process, and again on Foot Tàiyīn, 1 cone each.

衍義

（一）蛇蛻和豬頰車中髓傅頂，開發風氣於上，
　　　取髓以通其腦，單用豬頰車髓亦得。

（二）腦長不合，明系風寒痰氣襲入，故用薑、
　　　半開痰，芎、辛散風，桂心、烏頭辟除腦
　　　戶中邪氣。

（三）生蟹足散血續筋，白薟散結解毒。

（四）細辛、姜、桂能開發腦戶風寒，而不致於
　　　腦長，知無痰濕，故不用半夏。

（五）其風寒之邪本淺，故不用川芎。

Treatments for Skull Problems *Yǎn Yì* (Expanded Meaning)

(1) When spread on the vertex of the head, a mixture of *shétuì* and the marrow from the inside of a pig's lower jaw opens up and effuse wind qì in the upper body. We choose the marrow to open up the flow to the patient's brain. It is also possible to use the marrow from the inside of a pig's lower jaw on its own.

(2) A brain that is growing and failing to close up is clearly tied to an invasion of wind-cold phlegm qì. Therefore we use *shēngjiāng* and *bànxià* to open up the phlegm; *xiōngqióng* and *xìxīn* to dissipate the wind; and *guìxīn* and *wūtóu* to eliminate evil qì from within Nǎohù ("Brain Door").[27]

(3) Raw crab legs dissipate blood and thread together the sinews, while *báiliǎn* dissipates bindings and resolves toxin.

(4) *Xìxīn*, *gānjiāng*, and *guìxīn* are able to open up and effuse wind cold through Nǎo Hù. Since [the particular condition for which Sān Wù Xìxīn Fū Fāng is indicated] has not lead to an elongated brain, we know that there is no phlegm-damp present. Therefore we do not use *bànxià*.

(5) Since the evil of wind-cold has a shallow root, we therefore do not [need to] use *chuānxiōng*.

---

27 I have chosen to translate 腦戶 *nǎo hù* literally, but it also refers to the acumoxa point that is now identified as GV-17. My reason for the literal translation here and below is that the expression here seems to imply more than just a reference to a location. It appears important that the location is the entrance to the brain, the place where the pathogens related to this set of symptoms enter and exit.

（六）骨力猶能任身，故不用烏頭。

（七）風入系頭既久，故不用生薑而用乾姜，佐桂心以溫腦戶，即前半夏熨湯之變法。

（八）防風治惡風風邪，柏子仁除風濕潤燥，用白芨袪賊風痱緩，總皆療腦風藥。

（九）用豬牙中髓通腦氣於上，以無風毒，故無取於蛇蛻。

Commentary on Skull Problems *Yǎn Yì* ◂ **Sabine Wilms**

My translation of 痱緩 *féi huǎn* is based on the fact that *féi* here clearly does not refer to the skin condition translated by Wiseman in English as "prickly heat" (in which case the character is pronounced in the fourth tone, as *fèi*), but to what Wiseman translates as "disablement." According to the *Shénnóng Běncǎo Jīng*, *báijī* "governs welling-abscesses, malign sores, and vanquished flat-abscesses, damaged yīn and dead flesh, evil qì in the stomach, and bandit wind, *féi*, slackness, and loss of use of [the limbs]." The *Zhū Bìng Yuán Hòu Lùn* (vol. 1, entry on 風痱 *fēng féi*, "Wind Féi") describes the condition as "no pain in the body, loss of use of the limbs, no confusion in the spirit and mind, loss of use in one shoulder. If the patient can still speak at times, wind *féi* is treatable. If he or she cannot speak, it is not treatable.

(6) Because the strength of the bones is still able to hold the body up, we do not [need to] use *wūtóu*.

(7) Since wind has entered and tied up the head already for a long time, we do not use *shēngjiāng* but use *gānjiāng*, assisted by *guìxīn* to warm Nǎo Hù. This formula is thus a transformation of the method of the previously discussed Bànxià Yùn Tāng.

8) *Fángfēng* treats malign wind and wind evil; *bǎizǐrén* eliminates wind-damp and moistens dryness. We use *báijī* [because it] dispels bandit wind and *féi* disablement and slackness. All of these [substances] are medicinals that cure brain wind.

(9) The use of the marrow from inside a pig's teeth[28] opens up the flow of qì into the upper body. Based on the fact that there is no wind toxin present [in the conditions indicated in this formula], [the formula] does not include *shétuì*.

---

28 I read 牙 *yá* here as an abbreviation for 牙車 *yá chē*, meaning "lower jaw."

治小兒狐疝，傷損生癩方。

Commentary IX.9.a ◆ Sabine Wilms

狐疝 *hú shàn*: I have resisted the temptation of translating this evocative term quite literally as "foxy mounting" and instead have chosen the less colorful but more descriptive term "Fox Protrusion." *Hú shàn* is a technical term that refers to a protrusion of the contents of the lower abdomen into the scrotum, manifesting as a bulge in the groin that sometimes appears and sometimes retracts on its own or can be pushed back in by the patient when lying down. As such, it can be equated with the condition of inguinal hernia in biomedicine. Like a fox that is hiding in its den at night and emerges into plain sight during the day, this protrusion can be pushed back inside the body when the patient is lying down but will drop back down when the patient is standing up. For more information on *shàn*, see, for example, the discussion of 疝氣 *shàn qì* in the *Yī Zōng Jīn Jiàn*. The earliest medical text to describe Fox Protrusion is the *Língshū*. In volume 47, it is related to an abnormally low position of the kidney: "When the kidney is [abnormally] low, there is pain in the lumbus and coccyx and the patient is unable to look up or bend down. This produces Fox Protrusion" (腎下則腰尻痛，不可以俛仰，為狐疝). Somewhat similar to the associations of the English term "foxy," foxes are in Chinese culture associated with mischievousness and deviousness, especially when they shape-shift into beautiful maidens who seduce and ruin credulous young scholars. It is therefore no coincidence that a condition of the genital region is associated with the fox. Based on the etymology of the second character, 疝 *shàn*, which is a combination of the disease radical with the character for "mountain" (山), Wiseman translates it as "mounting." Nevertheless, the term has nothing to do with the action of "mounting" but merely refers to the mountain-like appearance of the protrusion.

IX.9 Problems with the Genitalia[29]

IX.9.a Formulas for Fox Protrusion and Testicular Bulging

Unnamed Formula
Indication
A formula for small children, to treat Fox Protrusion and the formation of testicular bulging as the result of injury

---

29   While some formulas in the section below are clearly gender-specific by referring to conditions of the testicles, others, such as genital sores, appear to be addressing conditions in girls as well. Somewhat confusingly, male-specific formulas are interspersed with ungendered ones in this single section and are not specifically differentiated by gender in the original text.

Commentary IX.9.a ✍ Sabine Wilms

癀 *tuí*: Wiseman translates this disease name quite literally as "prominence" or "bulging." The two characters 癀 and 㿗, both pronounced *tuí*, are used interchangeably in early sources, so should be translated with a single term here. According to the main entry on this disease in vol. 34 of the *Zhū Bìng Yuán Hòu Lùn*, "Testicular bulging manifests with swollen and enlarged testicles. Sometimes, there are short periods of remission, and when the remission times are over, [the testicles] grow larger than normal. The condition erupts after taxation, cold, yīn [weather conditions] and rain, and when it erupts, it causes hypertonicity in the lumbus and back of such a person, generalized aversion to cold, and sinking heaviness in the bones and joints. This disease is caused by injury to the kidney. The Foot Shàoyīn channel is the vessel of the kidney and its qì descends into the genitals. The genitals are the gathering place of the ancestral sinews and where yīn qì collects. Taxation damage or lifting heavy objects has damaged the Shàoyīn channel, and its qì rushes downward into the genitals. Qì becomes distended and does not flow through, therefore generating bulging testicles." In the pediatric section of the *Zhū Bìng Yuán Hòu Lùn*, vol. 50, the condition is further explained: "Testicular bulging is qì binding and [causing] swelling and enlargement in the testicles. When small children suffer from this condition, in most cases it is due to crying and anger and to pushing up the chest without stopping. This stirs up yīn qì, and yīn qì strikes, binding and gathering without scattering."

桂心	十八銖
地膚子	二兩半
白朮	一兩十八銖

（一）上三味，末之，以蜜和丸。

（二）白酒服如小豆七丸，日三。亦治大人。

又方

芍藥	各十八銖
茯苓	
防葵	各半兩
大黃	
半夏	各六銖
桂心	
蜀椒	

（一）上七味，末之，蜜和。

（二）服如大豆一丸，日五服，可加至三丸。

Ingredients

guìxīn	18 *zhū*
dìfùzǐ	2.5 *liǎng*
báizhú	1 *liǎng*, 18 *zhū*

Preparation

(1) Pulverize the three ingredients above and combine with honey to form pills.

(2) Take seven pills the size of mung beans in white liquor, three times a day. This formula also treats adults.

Another formula

Ingredients

sháoyào	18 *zhū* each
fúlíng	
*fángkuí**	0.5 *liǎng* each
dàhuáng	
bànxià	6 *zhū* each
guìxīn	
shǔjiāo	

Editorial comment: Another version has *fángfēng* here.

Preparation

(1) Pulverize the seven ingredients above and combine with honey [to form pills].

(2) Take one pill the size of a soy bean per dose, five doses per day. This dosage can be increased to three pills.

五等丸

治小兒陰偏大，又卵核堅癩方。

黃柏	
香豉	
牡丹	各二兩
防風	
桂心	

（一）上五味，末之，蜜丸如大豆。

（二）兒三歲飲服五丸，加至十丸。

（三）兒小以意酌量，著乳頭上服之。

IX.9.b Wǔ Děng Wán (Five Equals Pill)

Indication

A formula for small children, to treat unilateral enlargement of a testicle[30] as well as hardness and bulging of the testicles.

Ingredients

huángbò	
xiāngchǐ	
mǔdān	2 *liǎng* each
fángfēng	
guìxīn	

Preparation

(1) Pulverize the five ingredients above and form honey pills the size of soy beans.

(2) For a child of three *suì*, administer five pills per dose in liquid. The dosage can be increased up to ten pills.

(3) For a smaller child, use your discretion to determine the dosage. Administer [the medicine] by placing it on the nipple of the [mother's] breast.

---

30 While the source text does not specify that this condition only applies to male children, as implied by my translation of the originally non-gendered 陰 *yīn*, which can also be translated as "genitals," the placement of the formula in the present context, as well as the following symptom, which refers to the male testicle, have caused me to translate it as such here.

治小兒卵腫方。

取雞翅六莖，燒作灰服之，隨卵左右取翮。

治小兒癩方。

蜥蜴一枚，燒末，酒服之。

IX.9.c Formula for Swelling of the Testicles

Indication

A formula for small children, to treat swelling of the testicles.

Ingredients and Preparation

Take six chicken wings[31] and char them into ashes. Administer this orally. Choose left or right wings in accordance with the side that the enlarged testicle is on.[32]

IX.9.d Formula for Testicular Bulging

Indication

A formula for small children, to treat testicular bulging.

Ingredients and Preparation

Take a single lizard, char it into ashes, pulverize it, and have the patient ingest it in liquor.

---

31   In the *Yǎn Yì* commentary on this formula (translated below), the character 翅 *chì* ("wing") is replaced with the more specific character 翮 *hé*, meaning "quill." Given the context and the possible intention of the formula to lift up the swelling by means of something that is light enough to be blown about by wind, it seems more likely that this formula does in fact recommend to char chicken feathers instead of the whole wings. Another interesting side comment: The choice of chicken here might be related to the fact that the character used for "testicle," 卵 *luǎn*, literally means "egg."

32   Editorial comment: The version of this formula in the *Gǔjīn Lù Yàn* states: "It treats a testicle that is enlarged like a dipper."

衍義

（一）癪是濕熱阻積，滲入經隧之患。

（二）蜥蜴能吐雹祈雨，為利水破結之峻藥。

（三）《外臺》、《千金》恆用之。

治小兒氣癪方。

土瓜根
芍藥
當歸

上三味，各一兩，咬咀，以水二升，煮取一升，服五合，日二。

> ## Treatment of Testicular Bulging *Yǎn Yì* (Expanded Meaning)
>
> (1) Testicular bulging is a disorder caused by damp-heat obstructing and accumulating, and then percolating into the channels and tunnels.
>
> (2) Lizard [as a medicinal substance] is able to "vomit up hail and pray for rain."[33] It constitutes a harsh medicinal for disinhibiting water and breaking up bindings.
>
> (3) The *Wàitái Mìyào* and *Qiānjīn Fāng* constantly use it.
>
> ---
>
> 33 吐電祈雨 *tù báo qí yǔ*: This is a reference to a legend, according to which there once was a lizard on Mount Sòng that was several hundred years old. After inhaling water, it immediately spit it back out as blocks of ice, and then transformed the sound of thunder to cause rain and hail to fall from the sky.

IX.9.e Formulas for Qì Bulging

Unnamed Formula
Indication
A formula for small children, to treat qì bulging [of the testicles].

Ingredients

tǔguāgēn
sháoyào
dāngguī

Preparation
Pound 1 *liǎng* each of the three ingredients above and decoct in 2 *shēng* of water until reduced to 1 *shēng*. Take 5 *gě* per dose, two doses per day.

又方

（一）三月上除日，取白頭翁根搗之。

（二）隨偏處敷之，一宿作瘡，二十日愈。

灸足厥陰大敦，左灸右，右灸左，各一壯。

Another Formula

(1) On the "Elimination Day" of the third month,[34] take the root of *báitóuwēng* and crush it.

(2) Spread [the medicine] on the side where [the bulge] is located. After one night, a sore will have formed. After twenty days, the patient will have recovered.

IX.9.f Moxibustion Method

A Formula for Qì Bulging

Burn moxa on Dàdūn[35] on the Foot Juéyīn channel. If [the condition affects] the left, apply moxa to the right side; if [the condition affects] the right, apply moxa to the left, 1 cone each.

---

34 除日 *chú rì*: This expression denotes a certain lucky day that occurs in regular intervals in accordance with the lunar calendar. It is named such because it is an auspicious day for "eliminating" the old, and therefore by implication also for getting rid of pathologies like the testicular bulging addressed in this formula.

35 This is equivalent to the modern point LV-1, "Large Pile."

治小兒陰瘡方。

以人屎灰敷之，又狗屎灰敷之，又狗骨灰敷之，
又馬骨末敷之，皆可敷之。

Commentary IX.9.g ◄ Sabine Wilms

See *Zhū Bìng Yuán Hòu Lùn* vol. 40 for the main entry on
this condition, and vol. 50 specifically for the pediatric condition. The entry on "genital sores" in vol. 40 in the section
on the "Miscellaneous Disorders of Women," describes this
condition as follows: "Women's genital sores are caused by
worms feeding. The three worms and the nine worms in the
intestinal space become active and stir because of vacuity
in the *zàng* organs. When the force of the worms is slight, it
results in itching. When it is serious, it results in pain." The
entry on "Genital Swelling and the Formation of Sores" in
the pediatric section states: "In small children, heat in the
lower burner causes heat qì to surge against the genitals,
and the tip of the genitals suddenly becomes swollen and
shut, so the child is unable to urinate. Next, this causes the
formation of sores. It is commonly said that this is due to ash
and fire in the urine." Unlike the preceding formulas in section nine, this entire subsection on "Genital Sores" appears
to be addressing the condition in both boys and girls.

IX.9.g Formula for Genital Sores

Unnamed Formula

Indication

A formula for small children, to treat genital sores.

Preparation

Take human feces and char into ashes. Spread this on [the sores]. You can also use the ashes from [charred] dog feces or dog bones and spread that [on the sores]. Or you can pulverize horse bones and spread those on. All of these substances can be spread [on the sores].

治小兒歧股間連陰囊生瘡，汁出，先癢後痛，十
日五日自瘥，或一月或半月複發，連年 不瘥方。

灸瘡，搔去痂，帛拭令乾，以蜜敷，更溲面作燒
餅，熟即以餳塗餅熨之，冷即止，再度瘥。

IX.9.h Moxibustion Method

Indication

A formula for small children, to treat the formation of sores in the area between the juncture of the thigh and the scrotum, with oozing of liquid and first itching and then pain, spontaneous remission after five to ten days, but in a month or half a month erupting again, continuing [like this] for year after year without healing.

Treatment

Burn moxa on the sores and then scratch them to remove the scabs. Wipe them dry with silk and then apply honey. In addition, urinate on flour and make a baked flat cake. When it is done, spread malt sugar on the cake and then apply [the cake] as a hot compress [to the sores]. When it has cooled off, stop. After two treatments, recovery will ensue.

治小兒陰腫方。

狐莖灸，搗末，酒服之。

又方
搗蕪菁敷上。

又方
豬屎五升，水煮沸，布裹安腫上。
又方
搗垣衣敷之。

又
以衣中白魚敷之。

又方
斫桑木白汁塗之。

IX.9.i Formulas for Genital Swelling

Unnamed Formula
Indication
A formula for small children, to treat genital swelling.

Ingredients and Preparation
Roast a fox penis and pound it into a powder. Ingest it [mixed with] liquor.

Another Formula
Pound *wújīng* and spread it on [the sores].

Another Formula
Take 5 *shēng* of pig manure and decoct it in water, bringing it to a boil. Wrap it in cloth and press it on the swollen [area].

Another Formula
Pound moss from under old walls and apply that.

Another
You can also use silverfish and spread that on.

Another Formula
Crush mulberry wood into small pieces, take the white liquid, and spread it on.

衍義

（一）狐疝雖寒熱不同，一皆屬於肝經，故首推桂心通肝散經，白朮安脾逐濕，地膚專利小便，以泄濕熱也。

（二）又方芍藥、茯苓疏肝家濕熱，防葵、大黃泄疝瘕結熱，半夏一味專理痰濕，桂心、川椒開肝脾之向導。

（三）五等丸專主濕熱偏墜，黃柏清熱燥濕，防、豉散下焦風，牡丹和下焦血。

（四）桂心為熱因熱用之向導。

（五）雞屬巽走肝，六翮又為風之所發，專主風襲肝經之疝。

Treatments of Problems with the Genitalia *Yǎn Yì* (Expanded Meaning)

(1) Even though Fox Protrusion differs based on [whether it is related to] cold or heat, it is always associated with the liver channel. Therefore the first ingredient [in the formula IX.9.a above to treat it] is *guìxīn* to open up the flow to the liver and dissipate the channel. *Báizhú* quiets the spleen and dispels dampness, while d*ifùzǐ* specifically disinhibits urination. In this way, the formula drains damp-heat.

(2) In the next formula, *sháoyào* and *fúlíng* course damp-heat from the home of the liver; *fángkuí* and *dàhuáng* drain genital protrusions, conglomerations, and heat binds; the single ingredient *bànxià* specifically rectifies phlegm-damp, and *guìxīn* and *chuānjiāo* lead the way in opening up the liver and spleen.

(3) Wǔ Děng Wán is indicated specifically for damp-heat with unilateral sagging [of a single testicle]. *Huángbò* clears heat and dries dampness, *fángfēng* and *xiāngchǐ* dissipate wind from the lower burner, and *mǔdān* harmonizes blood in the lower burner.

(4) *Guìxīn* leads the way by means of the principle "using heat to treat heat."

(5) Chicken is associated with gently blowing through[36] the liver, and six quills [in particular] are something that [can be] lifted up by wind. [This substance] is specifically indicated for protrusions due to wind assailing the liver channel.

---

36 巽 *xùn*: This is a fairly obscure character that is associated with the *Yìjīng* hexagram for Wind. It describes the action or nature of wind, its ability to reach everywhere, whether in nature as external wind or in the human body as its internal equivalent. I have therefore translated it somewhat freely as "blowing through.")

（六）土瓜根散血，歸、芍和血，專主瘀血凝滯
之疝。

（七）白頭翁通風逐血，專主少陽、陽明風熱固
結之疝。

（八）股瘡灸之不瘥，取蜜以潤血燥，麵餅乘熱
以餳塗熨，取以助肝氣也。

（九）狐莖常縮入腹，達肝最捷，同氣相感之妙
用也。

（十）桑汁塗風熱，蕪菁薄熱腫。

（十一）垣衣傅熱毒。

（十二）衣魚散風腫。

（十三）豬矢解蘊蒸之熱也。

(6) *Tǔguāgēn* dissipates blood while *dāngguī* and *sháoyào* harmonize the blood. [This formula] thus is specifically indicated for genital protrusion due to static blood congealing and stagnating.

(7) *Báitóuwēng* opens up the movement of wind and expels blood. It is specifically indicated for genital protrusion that is related to wind heat in Shàoyáng and Yángmíng solidifying and binding.

(8) If you fail to cure sores on the thigh by means of moxibustion, take honey to moisten blood dryness. Wheat flour cake overcomes heat, when used as a hot compress on top of an application of malt sugar. These ingredients are chosen to assist liver qì.

(9) Fox penis always causes retraction back into the abdomen and is most nimble at reaching the liver. It is an ingenious application of the principle "identical qì respond to each other."

(10) Mulberry juice is spread on [to treat] wind heat, while *wújīng* is applied thinly [to treat] heat swelling.

(11) Moss from under walls is applied [to treat] heat toxin.

(12) Silverfish dissipate wind swelling.

(13) Pig manure is [used to] resolve brewing and steaming heat.

治小兒陰瘡方。

取狼牙濃煮汁洗之。

又方
黃連、胡粉等分，以香脂油和，敷之。

IX.10 Additional Genital Problems

IX.10.a Formulas for Genital Sores

Unnamed Formula
Indication
A formula for small children, to treat genital sores.

Ingredients and Preparation
Take *lángyá*[37] and simmer the concentrated juice. Wash [the sores] with the liquid.

Another Formula
Take equal amounts of *huánglián* and *húfěn*, mix with balsam oil and spread it on [the sores].

---

37   The present instructions do not specify whether the formula calls for the foliage or the root, both of which are used traditionally in Chinese medicine. My guess is that this information might have been considered irrelevant. As an "appended formula" (附方 *fù fāng*) in the entry on *lángyá* in the *Běncǎo Gāngmù* explains, "In the winter, use the root; in the summer, use the [fresh] foliage."

治小兒核腫，壯熱有實方。

甘遂	各十八銖
青木香	
石膏	
麝香	三銖
大黃	各一兩
前胡	
黃芩	半兩
甘草	十八銖

（一）上八味，㕮咀，以水七升，煮取一升九
合。

（二）每服三合，日四夜二。

小兒陰腫，灸大敦七壯。

IX.10.b Formula for Genital Nodes and Swelling[38]

Indication

A formula for small children, to treat nodes and swelling with vigorous heat [effusion] and the presence of repletion.

Ingredients

gānsuì	
qīngmùxiāng	18 *zhū* each
shígāo	
shèxiāng	3 *zhū*
dàhuáng	
qiánhú	1 *liǎng* each
huángqín	0.5 *liǎng*
gāncǎo	18 *zhū*

Preparation

(1) Pound the eight ingredients above and decoct in 7 *shēng* of water until reduced to 1 *shēng* and 9 *gě*.

(2) Take 3 *gě* per dose, four times a day and twice at night.

IX.10.c Moxibustion Method

For swelling of the genital area in small children, burn seven cones of moxa on Dàdūn.

---

38 An editorial comment in the *Rénmín Wèishēng* edition explains 核腫 *hé zhǒng* as a pathological condition caused by damp-heat pouring downward, causing qì stagnation and blood stasis and manifesting in swollen and enlarged node-like testicles. Nevertheless, the editors offer no reference for this interpretation and I therefore have chosen to translate the two characters literally in the Indications below. In other contexts, this combination of symptoms can just as well refer to a condition in the breasts, throat, or anywhere else. Based on the present context, however, it is most likely that this formula refers specifically to the formation of swelling and nodes in the genital area, but not necessarily only to male testicles.

鱉頭丸

治小兒積冷久下，瘥後餘脫肛不瘥，腹中冷，肛中疼痛，不得入者方。

死鱉頭	二枚，炙令焦
小蝟皮	一枚，炙令焦
磁石	四兩
桂心	三兩

（一）上四味，末之，蜜丸如大豆。

（二）兒三歲至五歲，服五丸至十丸，日三。兒大以意加之。

IX.10.d Biētóu Wán (Turtle's Head Pill)

Indication

A formula for small children, to treat long-term accumulation of cold that has been [eliminated by] moving it downwards. After the cure, [the patient is now suffering from] anal desertion[39] that is not healing, with cold inside the abdomen, pain inside the anus, and inability to reinsert [the prolapsed rectum].[40]

Ingredients

biētóu, dead	2 heads, roasted until scorched
wèipí	1 small one, roasted until scorched
císhí	4 *liǎng*
guìxīn	3 *liǎng*

Preparation

(1) Pulverize the four ingredients above and form honey pills the size of soy beans.

(2) For a child between three and five *suì*, give five to ten pills per dose, three times a day. For an older child, increase the dosage at your discretion.

---

39   This is the literal translation of 脫肛 *tuō gāng*, more commonly and perhaps elegantly translated as "prolapse of the rectum." I am intentionally leaving it literal here to emphasize the relationship to the "desertion of kidney qì" (腎氣之脫 *shèn qì zhī tuō*) mentioned in the *Yǎn Yì* explanation below.

40   I have chosen to simply translate this line as literally as possible. While modern critical editions all follow the wording and punctuation above, the *Yǎn Yì* edition instead says: "A formula for small children, to treat accumulations of cold that could not be cured by moxibustion, afterwards with prolapse of the rectum... (。。。積冷灸不瘥，後餘脫肛。。。). My interpretation of the last phrase in this line, literally "inability to enter," is based on a similar use of 入 *rù* in the moxibustion method below in line IX.11.a.

衍義

（一）狼牙殺蟲止痛。

（二）黃連、胡粉解熱收濕。

（三）青木香、前胡下結氣，甘草、石膏化結熱，大黃、黃芩、甘遂瀉濕熱，麝香開關竅。

（四）鱉頭收肝氣之緩，磁石固腎氣之脫，桂心散肝血之滯，猬皮破膀胱瘀積也。

小兒脫肛，灸頂上旋毛中三壯，即入。

又

灸尾翠骨三壯。

又

灸臍中隨年壯。

> **Treatments for Additional Genital Problems *Yǎn Yì* (Expanded Meaning)**
>
> (1) *Lángyá* kills bugs and stops pain.
>
> (2) *Huánglián* and *húfěn* resolve heat and astringe dampness.
>
> (3) *Qīngmùxiāng* and *qiánhú* move bound qì downward; *gāncǎo* and *shígāo* transform bound heat; *dàhuáng*, *huángqín*, and *gānsuì* drain damp-heat; and *shèxiāng* opens up closed orifices.
>
> (4) *Biētóu* contracts the laxness of liver qì; *císhí* secures the desertion of kidney qì; *guìxīn* dissipates the stagnation of liver blood; and *wèipí* breaks stasis accumulations in the urinary bladder.

IX.11 Moxibustion for Anal Desertion

For anal desertion in small children, burn three cones of moxa on the vertex of the head in the center where the hair curls. Then [you will be able to] reinsert [the prolapsed rectum into the anus].

Another [Moxibustion Treatment]

Burn three cones of moxa on Wěicuìgǔ.[41]

Another [Moxibustion Treatment]

Burn moxa in the center of the navel, the number of cones being equal to the child's age.

---

41 Literally, these three characters mean either "tail kingfisher bone" (as it is usually translated in modern medical literature) or, more likely, "bone by a bird's tail," based on the fact that 翠 can be read as 膵, which means the "meat on a bird's tail." This is a non-channel point described in the *Tàipíng Shèng Huì Fāng* as located 3 *cùn* above the coccyx and indicated for "pediatric *gān* dysentery, anal desertion and emaciation, thirst with intake of fluids, physical frailness and haggardness, and whatever conditions physicians are unable to cure." In modern medical literature, it is identified as GV-1.

治小兒痚濕瘡方。

鐵衣著下部中，即瘥。

治小兒久痢膿濕䘌方。

艾葉五升，以水一斗，煮取一升半，分為三服。

Commentary IX.12.B ↩ Sabine Wilms

䘌 *nì* is a pathology that is discussed by Cháo Yuánfāng in the *Zhū Bìng Yuán Hòu Lùn* in great detail (see volume 18). Arising after incorrect or insufficient treatment of a variety of other conditions, it is caused by a weakness in the spleen and stomach, which is allowing damp-heat to invade and take advantage of the vacuity of right qì. Damp *nì* in particular is characterized by the following etiology: "The weakness and vacuity of the spleen and stomach is allowing water-damp to invade, causing stirring of bugs inside the abdomen. When they invade the food, they form *nì* worms. Usually related to incessant diarrhea, possibly after seasonal disease, it is caused by invading heat binding internally. It manifests with inability to eat and drink, desire to sleep, slight heat effusion, heaviness in the joints and bones, pervasive whiteness on the tongue, and fine millet-like sores. If there are sores forming on the upper lips, this means that the worms are eating the five viscera, causing heart vexation and oppression. If there are sores forming on the lower lips, this means that the worms are eating the lower part of the body, resulting in erosion and openness of the anus…"

IX.12 Problems with Dampness

IX.12.a Formula for *Gān* Dampness

Indication

A formula for small children, to treat *gān* dampness sores.

Ingredients and Preparation

Place rust in contact with the patient's private parts, and recovery will ensue.

IX.12.b Formula for Dysentery with Damp *Nì* Worms

Indication

A formula for small children, to treat chronic dysentery with pus and damp *nì* worms.

Ingredients and Preparation

Take 5 *shēng* of *àiyè* and decoct in 1 *dǒu* of water until reduced to 1.5 *shēng*. Divide into three doses.

蠹

治小兒疳瘡方。

以豬脂和胡粉敷之，五六度。

又方

嚼麻子敷之，日六七度。

又方

羊膽二枚，和醬汁於下部灌之。豬脂亦佳。

Commentary IX.12.c ❧ Sabine Wilms

疳 gān: Sometimes identified too narrowly with "rickets," this term can perhaps be rendered best in English as "infantile malnutrition," because it is a condition of early childhood that is related to malnutrition. In Qián Yǐ's famous pediatrics text *Xiǎoér Yào Zhèng Zhí Jué* (小兒藥証直訣) from the Sòng period, it is defined as "always a disease of the spleen and stomach, it is caused by a lack of fluids" (皆脾胃病,亡津液之所作也). In volume 50 of the *Zhū Bìng Yuán Hòu Lùn*, we find an entry on "*gān* dampness sores" that explains the condition as follows: "The disease of *gān* dampness is in most cases caused by chronic diarrhea, causing vacuity and weakness of the spleen and stomach, and stirring of worms in the gastrointestinal area, which invade and erode the five *zàng* organs and cause the person to suffer from heart vexation and oppression. When the erosion takes place in the upper body, sores form on the mouth, nose, or gums. When it takes place in the lower body, the anus is damaged by putrefaction. This condition is always difficult to treat. Perhaps it was caused by chronic diarrhea, perhaps by heat in the *zàng* organs and somnolence, perhaps by an excessive appetite for eating sweet delicacies. In all cases, [these factors] cause the worms to stir and subsequently form this disease." It is no coincidence that the character for *gān* consists of the disease radical in combination with the character 甘, meaning "sweet" and pronounced *gān* as well.

IX.12.c Formulas for *Gān* Sores

Indication
A formula to treat *gān* sores in small children.[42]

Ingredients and Preparation
Take lard and mix it with *húfěn*. Apply this [to the sores] five or six times.

Another Formula
Chew hemp seeds and spread them on [the sores], six or seven times a day.

Another Formula
Take two gallbladders from sheep or goats, mix with pickling juice, and pour onto the private parts. Lard is also excellent.

42　疳瘡 *gān chuāng*: The *Yǎn Yì* edition has 疳瘧 *gān nüè* "*gán* malaria" here instead, which does exist as a pathological condition. I consider the earlier *Sūn Zhēn Rén* edition to be much more reliable, however, as a guide to textual accuracy, and therefore choose to follow that edition, which concurs with the received version in having "*gān* sores" here instead.

Commentary IX.12.c ᴥ **Julian Scott**

Gān 'malnutrition' is a further development of accumulation disorder. There is usually heat and emaciation going with it. But you do get sores even with accumulation disorder.

治濕瘡方。

濃煎地榆汁洗浴，每日二度。

小兒疳濕瘡，灸第十五椎挾脊兩旁七壯，未瘥，加七壯。

IX.12.d Formula for Dampness Sores

Indication

A formula to treat dampness sores.

Ingredients and Preparation

Simmer *dìyú* juice down until concentrated and bathe [the patient] with this, twice each day.

IX.12.e Moxibustion for *Gān* Dampness

For *gān* dampness sores in small children, burn seven cones of moxa on both sides of the spine by the fifteenth vertebra. If the patient fails to recover, use an additional seven cones.

除熱結腸丸

斷小兒熱，下黃赤汁沫，及魚腦雜血，肛中瘡
爛，坐蠶生蟲方。

Commentary IX.12.f✒ Sabine Wilms

坐蠶 *zuò nì*: I am not sure about the meaning of "sitting" here,
but *nì* is a pathology defined as follows in the *Zhū Bìng Yuán
Hòu Lùn*, volume 18: "The disease of damp *nì* is caused by vacuity
and weakness in the spleen and stomach that is then exploited
by water damp. Worms stir inside the abdomen, invade and feed
to form *nì*. In most cases, it is caused to incessant diarrhea or to
intrusive heat after seasonal disease binding in the abdomen.
It manifests with inability to drink and eat, absentmindedness
and somnolence, continuous mild heat, heaviness in the bones
and joints, lusterless teeth, complete whiteness on the surface of
the tongue, and fine sores like millet grains. If the sores form on
the upper lip, this means that the worms are eating the five *zàng*
organs, which results in heart vexation and oppression. If the
sores form on the lower lip, this means that the worms are eating
the lower body, which results in putrefaction and opening of the
anus. In severe cases, all the internal organs get eaten and sores

IX.12.f Chú Rè Jié Cháng Wán (Heat-Eliminating Intestines-Binding Pill)

Indication

A formula to interrupt small children's heat [that manifests] with discharge of yellow or red foamy liquid and [a substance like] fish-brain mixed with blood, sores and putrefaction in the anus, and sitting *nì* generating worms.

Commentary IX.12.f ⁕ Sabine Wilms (continued)

form everywhere above and below the teeth on the gums, the color of the teeth is purplish black, and [the patient suffers from] diarrhea of blood and dampness, which is due to water qì." In the following section, Cháo Yuánfāng explains that harmonious functioning of the spleen and stomach is essential for transforming the essence of food and drink into blood and qi to nourish the internal organs. When the spleen and stomach are weakened, however, earth qì is debilitated and can contract cold or be damaged by heat, resulting in diarrhea. As the result of vacuity heat in the intestines and stomach, worms are able to thrive and consume the internal organs, eventually appearing in the mouth above and anus below. Over time, the worms consume the organs and thereby cause the patient's death as the result of bloody diarrhea. The *Zhū Bìng Yuán Hòu Lùn* discusses three subcategories of *nì* worms, namely dampness *nì* (related to the presence of dampness), heart *nì* (specifically affecting the heart and manifesting in heart vexation), and *gān nì* (associated with a predilection for eating sweets that has facilitated stirring of worms.

黃連	
柏皮	
苦參	
鬼臼	各半兩
獨活	
橘皮	
芍藥	
阿膠	

上八味，末之，以藍汁及蜜丸如小豆，日服三丸
至十丸。

Ingredients

huánglián	
bópí	
kǔshēn	
guǐjiù	0.5 *liǎng* each
dúhuó	
júpí	
sháoyào	
ējiāo	

Preparation

Pulverize the eight ingredients above and combine them with *lánzhī* and honey to make pills the size of mung beans. Each day, take three pills, [increasing the dosage to] up to ten pills.[43]

---

43 Editorial comment: In the winter, when no *lánzhī* is available, you can use 1 *gě* of the seeds, pestled and mixed with honey to form pills.

衍義

（一）疳瘡內蘊濕熱，外顯血燥，故用鐵衣以降
　　濕火。

（二）胡粉、豬脂兼濟，收濕潤燥之治。

（三）麻子專取潤燥。

（四）羊膽專取化熱。

（五）地榆散血止痛。

（六）艾葉溫血化䘌。

（七）結腸丸專泄濕熱，僅用鬼白以殺毒邪，獨
　　活以散風熱。

治小兒蚘蟲方。

楝木削上蒼皮，以水煮取汁飲之，量大小多少，
為此有小毒。

Dampness Formulas *Yǎn Yì* **Expanded Meaning**

(1) *Gān* sores are [a sign of] internally smoldering damp-heat, the external manifestation of blood dryness. Therefore the formula uses rust to downbear dampness and fire.

(2) *Húfěn* and lard provide simultaneous relief with a treatment of astringing dampness and moistening dryness

(3) *Mázǐ* is specifically chosen for its effect of moistening dryness.

(4) Goat or sheep gallbladder is specifically chosen for its effect of transforming heat.

(5) *Dìyú* dissipates blood and stops pain.

(6) *Àiyè* warms the blood and transforms *nì* worms.

(7) Jié Cháng Wán specifically drains damp-heat, using only *guǐjiù* to kill toxin evil and *dúhuó* to dissipate wind heat.

IX.13 Parasites

IX.13.a Formula for Roundworm

Indication

A formula for small children, to treat roundworm.

Ingredients and Preparation

Take chinaberry tree wood and shave off the grayish bark. Simmer it in water, then take the liquid and drink it. For the dosage, take the patient's age into account. This is because this formula is slightly toxic.

治小兒羸瘦有蛔蟲方。

藋蘆二兩，以水一升，米二合煮，取米熟去滓，
與服之。

又方
萹蓄三兩，水一升，煮取四合，分服之。搗汁服
亦佳。

又方

東引吳茱萸根白皮	四兩
桃白皮	三兩

上二味，咬咀，以酒一升二合，漬之一宿，漸與
服，取瘥。

又方
取豬膏服之。

IX.13.b Formulas for Emaciation Due to Roundworm

Unnamed Formula

Indication

A formula for small children, to treat marked emaciation [related to] the presence of roundworm.

Ingredients and Preparation

Take 2 *liǎng* of *guànlú* and simmer in 1 *shēng* of water with 2 *gě* of rice. When the rice is cooked, remove the dregs and have [the patient] ingest [the decoction].

Another Formula

Decoct 3 *liǎng* of *biānxù* in 1 *shēng* of water until reduced to 4 *gě*. Divide it into doses and have the patient ingest it. Pounding it and ingesting the juice is also excellent.

Another formula

Ingredients

wúzhūyú, the white skin of an eastward-leading root	4 *liǎng*
white skin [from the root of] a peach tree	3 *liǎng*

Ingredients and Preparation

Pound the two ingredients above and soak overnight in 1 *shēng* and 2 *gě* of liquor. Give this to the patient in small amounts to take internally, and recovery will ensue.

Another Formula

Get some lard and have the patient take this internally.[44]

---

44 Editorial comment: According to another version, this formula treats pinworm.

又方

搗槐子納下部中，瘥為度。

又方

楝實一枚納孔中。

治寸白蟲方。

東行石榴根一把，水一升，煮取三合，分服。

又方

桃葉搗絞取汁服之。

Another Formula

Pound *huáizĭ* and insert them into the anus,[45] Taking recovery as your measurement [that you can stop administering the medicine].[46]

Another Formula

Take one piece of *liànshí* and insert it into the opening [of the anus].[47]

IX.13.c Formulas for Inch Whiteworm[48]

Indication

A formula to treat inch whiteworm.

Ingredients and Preparation

Decoct one handful of eastward-growing *shíliúgēn* in 1 *shēng* of water until reduced to 3 *gě*. Divide into doses.

Another Formula

Pound leaves from a peach tree and wring them out to get the juice. Administer this orally.

---

45 Literally, the text says to insert them "into the lower section [of the body]."

46 Editorial comment: According to another version, this formula treats pinworm.

47 Editorial comment: According to another version, this formula treats pinworm.

48 寸白蟲 *cùn bái chóng*: I am following Wiseman in maintaining a literal translation of this term. It is most likely associated with tapeworm infestation in biomedical terms.

治小兒三蟲方。

| 雷丸 |
| 芎藭 |

上二味，各等分，為末。服一錢匕，日二。

治大便竟出血方。

（一）鱉頭一枚，炙令黄黑，末之。

（二）以飲下五分匕，多少量兒大小，日三服。

又方

燒甑帶末敷乳頭上，令兒飲之。

IX.13.d Formula for Worms

Indication

A formula for the three kinds of worms in small children.[49]

Ingredients

léiwán
xiōngqióng

Preparation

Take equal amounts of the two ingredients above and make a powder. Administer 1 *qián*-spoonful, twice a day.

IX.13.e Formulas for Bloody Stools

Indication

A formula to treat unexpected bloody discharge in the stools.

Ingredients and Preparation

(1) Roast one *biētóu* until it is yellowish black and pulverize it.

(2) Ingest a 5-*fēn* spoonful in liquid, adjusting the amount by the child's age, three doses a day.

Another Formula

Roast a steaming pot band[50] and pulverize it. Apply this to the nipple and have the child nurse from it.

---

49   According to the *Zhū Bìng Yuán Hòu Lùn*, the "three worms" is a reference to 長蟲*cháng chóng* ("longworms"), 赤蟲 *chì chóng* ("redworms"), and 蟯蟲 *náo chóng* ("pinworms").

50   See footnote 6 of this chapter on p. 345 for more on this medicinal ingredient.

又方

燒車缸一枚令赤，納一升水中，分二服。

衍義

（一）楝皮苦寒，治濕化蟲。

（二）蓳蘆涼潤，解毒清熱。

（三）萹蓄利水，治浸淫濕熱。

（四）桃皮殺蟲，茛根除濕。

（五）豬脂專引肛門蟯蟲。

（六）槐子專消大腸濕熱。

（七）楝實苦寒與楝皮同功。

（八）榴皮袪濕。

（九）桃葉化䘌。

（十）雷丸殺蟲，芍藥和血。

（十一）鱉頭收肛，專散肝經濕熱。

Another Formula

Roast a cart tire[51] until glowing red and place it in 1 *shēng* of water. Divide into two doses.

___

51 In early medieval China, these tires consisted of metal bands placed around wooden wheels.

Yǎn Yì (Expanded Meaning)

(1) *Liànpí* is bitter and cold. It treats dampness and transforms worms.

(2) *Guànlú* is cool and moistening. It resolves toxin and clears heat.

(3) *Biānxù* disinhibits water and treats wet spreading [sores] and damp-heat.

(4) Peach root bark kills worms, and *wúzhūyú* root eliminates dampness.

(5) Lard specifically draws pinworms to the anus.

(6) *Huáizǐ* specifically disperses damp-heat in the large intestine.

(7) *Liànshí* is bitter and cool and has the same medicinal effect as *liànpí*.

(8) *Shíliúpí* dispels dampness.

(9) *Táoyè* transforms *nì* worms.

(10) *Léiwán* kills worms, and *sháoyào* harmonizes the blood.

(11) *Biētóu* contracts the anus and specifically dissipates damp-heat in the liver channel.

治小兒尿血方。

（一）燒鵲巢灰，井花水服之。
（二）亦治夜尿床。

又方
尿血，灸第七椎兩旁各五寸，隨年壯。

衍義

小兒尿血多緣肝受風熱，不能藏血，故取久受風
氣之鵲巢燒服，以散肝風，風散則血自寧矣。

IX.14 Hematuria

Indication
A formula for small children, to treat hematuria.

Ingredients and Preparation
(1) Char a magpie's nest into ashes and have the patient ingest this in well flower water.

(2) This [formula] also treats bedwetting.

Another Formula
For hematuria, burn moxa [on a location] 5 *cùn* to both sides of the seventh vertebra, with the number of cones identical with the patient's age.

> ### Treatments for Hematuria *Yǎn Yì* (Expanded Meaning)
>
> In small children, hematuria is primarily caused by the contraction of wind heat in the liver, as the result of which it is unable to store the blood. Therefore we take a magpie's nest that has received wind qì for a long time, char it, and have the patient ingest it, to dissipate liver wind. Once the wind is dissipated, the blood will simply calm down on its own.

治小兒遺尿方。

瞿麥	
龍膽	各半兩
皂莢	
桂心	
雞腸草	一兩
車前子	一兩 六銖
石韋	半兩
人參	一兩

（一）上八味，末之，蜜丸。

（二）每食後服如小豆大五丸，日三，加至六七丸。

又方

小豆葉搗汁服。

Commentary IX.15.a ◆ Sabine Wilms

According to the *Zhū Bìng Yuán Hòu Lùn*, "Enuresis is caused by the presence of cold in the urinary bladder, which is preventing it from constraining water. The Foot Tàiyīn is the channel of the Bladder, while the Foot Shàoyīn is the channel of the Kidney. These two channels stand in an exterior-interior relationship to each other. The kidney governs water and kidney qì [is in charge of] downward movement and free flow to the genitals. Urine is the remainder of the fluids. The bladder is the *fǔ* organ of the fluids and when cold qì has weakened it, it is unable to constrain water. This is the cause of enuresis."

IX.15 Enuresis

IX.15.a Formulas for Enuresis

Unnamed Formula
Indication
A formula for small children, to treat enuresis.

Ingredients

qúmài	0.5 *liǎng* each
lóngdǎn	
zàojiá	
guìxīn,	
jīchángcǎo	1 *liǎng*
chēqiánzǐ	1 *liǎng* 6 *zhū*
shíwéi	0.5 *liǎng*
rénshēn	1 *liǎng*

Preparation
(1) Pulverize the eight ingredients above and form into honey pills.

(2) After each meal, take five pills the size of mung beans, three times a day. [If necessary,] increase the dosage to six or seven pills.

Another Formula
Crush the foliage of *xiǎodòu* [to gain] the juice and have the patient ingest that.

又方

燒雞腸末之，漿水服方寸匕，日三。

遺尿，灸臍下一寸半，隨年壯。

又

灸大敦三壯。亦治尿血。

Another Formula

Char chicken intestines[52] and pulverize them. Take a square-*cùn* spoonful in sour millet water, three times a day.[53]

IX.15.b Moxibustion for Enuresis

For enuresis, burn moxa [on a spot] 1.5 *cùn* below the navel, with the number of cones identical with the patient's age.

Another [Treatment]

Burn three cones of moxa on Dàdūn. This also treats hematuria.

---

52   In spite of the fact that the use of *jīchángcǎo* (literally, "chicken intestine herb") above might suggest that the present formula also calls for the herb, I have translated the term here literally as "chicken intestines" for several reasons: Most importantly, the medicinal use of chicken intestines for the treatment of enuresis has been recorded in materia medica literature throughout Chinese medical history, starting with the *Shénnóng Běncǎo Jīng*. Second, it is common to "char and pulverize" animal products but not simple herbs. And thirdly, if this formula were referring to the herb, it would most likely specify the herb by adding 草 *cǎo* ("herb") to make this clear, especially in the context of treating enuresis, for which the literal meaning of the term is specifically indicated while the herb is not.

53   Editorial comment: Another version states to ingest it while facing the Big Dipper.

衍義

（一）小兒遺尿多屬肝氣之熱，故用瞿麥、石韋、龍膽、雞腸、車前一派清熱利水之藥，兼桂心以司開關之權，人參以助清熱之力，皂莢以振滌垢之威，不使關閘有所阻積而失權度。

（二）小豆葉清熱，雞腸末利水，皆疏利九竅之品。

Commentary IX.15.b ๙ Julian Scott

The kind of enuresis Sūn Sīmiǎo is referring to is not the condition that is most commonly seen in the children of wealthy patients, who are more likely to suffer from cold and deficient conditions. The liver heat pattern discussed here is more common in the children of deprived and angry parents. It is interesting that he thinks it worthwhile to mention moxibustion for enuresis. This is because even in the heat pattern, the condition is often due to local weakness, which responds better to local treatment.

Treatments for Enuresis *Yǎn Yì* (Expanded Meaning)

(1) In small children, enuresis is associated in most cases with heat of liver qì. Therefore [the first formula above] uses *qúmài, shíwéi, lóngdǎn, jīchángcǎo,* and *chēqiánzǐ* from the single category of heat-clearing and water-disinhibiting medicinals. These ingredients are combined with *guìxīn* to supervise the authority of opening and closing, with *rénshēn* to assist the strength of clearing heat, and with *zàojiá* to arouse its might of sweeping away filth. In this way, we ensure that there are no obstructions or accumulations [to impair the functioning] of the sluice gates and that they do not lose their proper measure.

(2) *Xiǎodòu* foliage clears heat, and pulverized [charred] chicken intestines disinhibit water. Both of these ingredients are substances that course and disinhibit the nine orifices.

地膚子湯

治小兒熱毒入膀胱中，忽患小便不通，欲小便則
澀痛不出，出少如血，須臾復出方。

地膚子	各六銖
瞿麥	
知母	
黃芩	
枳實	
升麻	
葵子	
豬苓	
海藻	各三銖
橘皮	
通草	
大黃	十八銖

IX.16 Urination

IX.16.a Dìfūzǐ Tāng (Kochia Decoction)

Indication

A formula for small children, to treat heat toxin that has entered inside the urinary bladder. [The patient] suddenly suffers from urine failing to flow through or, whenever the patient is about to urinate, from unsmooth flow, pain, and either no discharge [of urine] at all or a scant discharge [of fluid] that resembles blood and after a moment another discharge.

Ingredients

dìfùzǐ	
qúmài	
zhīmǔ	
huángqín	
zhǐshí	6 *zhū* each
shēngmá	
kuízǐ	
zhūlíng	
hǎizǎo	
júpí	3 *zhū* each
tōngcǎo	
dàhuáng	18 *zhū*

（一）上十二味，㕮咀，以水三升，煮取一升。

（二）一日至七日兒，服一合，為三服。八日至
　　　十五日兒，一合半為三服。十六日至二十
　　　日兒，二合為三服。四十日兒以此為準。
　　　五十日以上、七歲以下，以意加藥益水。

治小兒淋方。

車前子一升，水二升，煮取一升，分服。

又方

煮冬葵子汁服之。

又方

取蜂房、亂髮燒灰，以水服一錢匕，日再。

Preparation

(1) Pound the twelve ingredients above and decoct in 3 *shēng* of water until reduced to 1 *shēng*.

(2) For a child one to seven days old, have them ingest 1 *gě* [per dose] and give three doses. For a child eight to fifteen days old, have them ingest 1.5 *gě* [per dose] and give three doses. For a child sixteen to twenty days old, have them ingest 2 *gě* [per dose] and give three doses. For a child forty days old, take this formula [above] as your precise dosage.[54] For a child between fifty days and seven *suì* old, use your discretion to increase the [amount of] medicinals and water.

IX.16.b Formulas for Strangury

Unnamed Formula

Indication

A formula for small children, to treat strangury.

Ingredients and Preparation

Decoct 1 *shēng* of *chēqiánzǐ* in 2 *shēng* of water until reduced to 1 *shēng* and divide into doses.

Another Formula

Decoct *dōngkuízǐ* and have the patient ingest the liquid.

Another Formula

Take *fēngfáng* and *luànfà* and char into ashes. Ingest a 1-*qián* spoonful in water, twice a day.

---

54 In other words, give the patient the full amount of medicine produced in one batch of the present formula above. The fact that you would still divide it up into three doses is obvious and therefore not stated explicitly.

治小兒小便不通方。

車前草	切，一升
小麥	一升

上二味，以水二升，煮取一升二合，去滓，煮粥服，日三四。

又方

冬葵子一升，以水二升，煮取一升，分服，入滑石末六銖。

衍義

（一）小兒腎氣完固，熱毒流入膀胱，自當專力苦寒，以利關竅，獨用升麻升舉上氣，海藻疏達下源，使熱泄水利，無複艱阻之慮矣。

（二）車前利水而不傷津，冬葵子利竅而兼活血。

IX.16.c Formulas for Stopped Urination

Unnamed Formula

A formula for small children, to treat failure of the urine to flow through.

Ingredients

chēqiáncǎo	chopped, 1 *shēng*
xiǎomài	1 *shēng*

Preparation

Of the two ingredients above, decoct [the herb] in 2 *shēng* of water until reduced to 1 *shēng* and 2 *gě*. Remove the dregs. Simmer [this decoction together with the *xiǎomài* to prepare] gruel and have the patient ingest that, three to four times a day.

Another Formula

Decoct 1 *shēng* of *dōngkuízǐ* in 2 *shēng* of water until reduced to 1 *shēng*. Divide into doses. Add 6 *zhū* of pulverized *huáshí*.

Treatments of Problems with Urination *Yǎn Yì* (Expanded Meaning)

(1) In small children, when kidney qì is already completely consolidated and then heat toxin flows into the urinary bladder, we should naturally focus our efforts specifically on bitter and cooling [medicinals], to disinhibit the orifices. Hence [the first formula above] merely uses *shēngmá* to lift up qì and *hǎizǎo* to course and outthrust the lower origin. This [approach] causes heat to be discharged and water to be disinhibited. As a result we will not have to worry about dangerous obstructions again.

(2) *Chēqiánzǐ* disinhibits water without damaging the fluids, while *dōngkuízǐ* disinhibits the orifices and at the same time quickens blood.

（三）蜂房、髮灰、善散膀胱瘀血。

（四）卷耳利水，同小麥益肝，煮粥以養胃氣，
　　　並杜虛熱之復擾。

（五）冬葵利竅活血，入滑石尤捷，與車前、小
　　　麥隱然有虛實之分。

(3) *Fēngfáng* and *luànfā* excel at dissipating static blood from the bladder.

(4) *Chēqiáncǎo*[55] disinhibits water and, just like *xiǎomài*, boosts the liver. Prepared as a gruel, [these ingredients] thereby have the effect of nurturing stomach qì and at the same time stopping the recurrent harassment by vacuity heat.

(5) *Dōngkuízǐ* disinhibits the orifices and vitalizes the blood. Adding *huáshí* makes [this formula] particularly fast-acting. In comparison with the combination of *chēqiánzǐ* and *xiǎomài* [in the previous formula], there is the subtle difference of [addressing] vacuity versus repletion.

---

55 The *Yǎn Yì* has here replaced the term *chēqiáncǎo* in the formula above with *juǎněr*. The original formula's use of Plantaginis Herba makes perfect sense in the current context since its traditional primary indication is indeed to disinhibit urination. While *juǎněr* is indeed a name that is sometimes used as a substitute to refer to *chēqiáncǎo*, it refers strictly speaking to a completely different plant, namely *Cerastium arvense* or, as already recorded in the *Ěryǎ* dictionary, to 蒼耳 *cāngěr* (*Xanthii Herba*), an herb that is indicated in the *Shénnóng Běncǎo Jīng* for wind in the head, cold pain, wind damp, impediment, and similar conditions. I have taken the liberty to correct this substitution here in the *Yǎn Yì*, because the commentary obviously refers to the medicinal ingredient used in the formula above for a gruel made with *xiǎomài*

治小兒吐血方。

燒蛇蛻皮末，以乳服之，並治重舌。

又方
取油三分，酒一分和之，分再服。

衍義

（一）小兒吐血，有毒熱，無虛寒，故宜去風解
　　　毒為務。

（二）蛇蛻燒灰，不特截風，兼能止血，血本肝
　　　經所藏也。

（三）其用香油解毒，必兼醇酒和血，總無藉於
　　　培養血氣。

IX.17 Vomiting Blood

Unnamed Formula

Indication

A formula for small children, to treat vomiting blood.

Ingredients and Preparation

Char *shétuìpí* and pulverize it. Have the patient ingest it with breast milk. This also treats double tongue.

Another Formula

Take 3 parts [sesame] oil and 1 part liquor and mix them together. Divide into two doses and have the patient ingest it.

Treatments for Vomiting Blood *Yǎn Yì* (Expanded Meaning)

(1) When small children vomit blood, this means the presence of toxic heat and the absence of vacuity cold. Therefore it is appropriate to focus treatment on getting rid of wind and resolving toxin.

(2) *Shétuìpí* charred into ashes not only interrupts wind but is able at the same time to stanch bleeding. Blood is originally a substance that is stored in the liver channel.

(3) The use of sesame oil here resolves toxin, but it must be combined with high-grade liquor to harmonize the blood, even if it does not rely on building up blood and qì.

治小兒鼻塞生息肉方。

通草	各一兩
細辛	

上二味，擣末，取藥如豆，著綿纏頭，納鼻中，
日二。

IX.18 Nose Problems

IX.18.a Formula for Nasal Congestion with Polyps

Indication

A formula for small children, to treat nasal congestion with the formation of polyps.

Ingredients

tōngcǎo	1 *liǎng* each
xìxīn	

Preparation

Pound the two ingredients above into a powder. Take a roughly bean-sized amount of the medicine, make it adhere to silk floss and coil it up into a head.[56] Insert it into the nose. [Apply this treatment] twice a day.

---

56   I read this line as instructing the doctor to dip the silk floss into the powdered herbs until it holds a roughly bean-sized amount and then to twist the silk floss into the shape of a "head." This bulge of silk floss with powdered herbs can then be inserted into the patient's nose as a way to have the patient absorb the medicine. Alternatively, you could read this line as telling the doctor to wind the string of silk floss around the patient's head, possibly as a way of attaching the silk to the young patient, and insert the end that is impregnated with the medicinals into the patient's nose. Given the fact that the herbs are prepared as a dry powder and that it doesn't seem safe or practical to tie a string of silk floss around a baby's head twice a day however, this interpretation makes a lot less sense to me.

治小兒鼻塞不通，濁涕出方。

杏仁半兩	
蜀椒	
附子	
細辛各六銖	

（一）上四味，咬咀，以醋五合，漬藥一宿。

（二）明旦以豬脂五合煎，令附子色黄，膏成，去滓。

（三）待冷以塗絮導鼻孔中，日再，兼摩頂上。

IX.18.b Formula for Nasal Congestion with Turbid Discharge

Indication

A formula for small children, to treat nasal congestion, complete blockage, and discharge of turbid snivel.

Ingredients

xìngrén	0.5 *liǎng*
shǔjiāo	
fùzǐ	6 *zhū* each
xìxīn	

Preparation

(1) Pound the four ingredients above. Soak the medicine in 5 *gě* of vinegar overnight.

(2) On the next day, simmer it in 5 *gě* of lard until the *fùzǐ* has turned yellow. This means that the salve is done. Remove the dregs.

(3) Wait to let it cool off, then spread it on silk wadding and insert it into the nostril. Apply two treatments a day. At the same time massage it into the vertex of the head.

衍義

（一）通草利竅散濕，細辛利竅散風。

（二）風散濕去則經脈條暢。

（三）何有窒塞息肉之患乎。

（四）杏仁下氣，川椒溫中，附子逐濕，細辛去風，皆利竅之品。

（五）其用醋者，藉以領諸藥入於肝經，且遏椒、附之性，緩行不以驟也。

Treatments for Nose Problems *Yǎn Yì* (Expanded Meaning)

(1) *Tōngcǎo* disinhibits the orifices and dissipates dampness, while *xìxīn* disinhibits the orifices and dissipates wind.

(2) When wind is dissipated and dampness removed, the channels will be smooth and free-flowing.

(3) How could any trouble with congestion and polyps remain?

(4) *Xìngrén* moves qì downward, *chuānjiāo* warms the center, *fùzǐ* expels dampness, and *xìxīn* removes wind. All of these are substances that disinhibit the orifices.

(5) The use of vinegar [in this formula] is for the purpose of leading all the medicinals into the liver channel while at the same time checking the [drastic] nature of *chuānjiāo* and *fùzǐ* and slowing down their movement to prevent them from "galloping."[57]

---

57 "Galloping" medicines are medicines that act too harshly and thereby threaten to damage the child's tender constitutional state.

治小兒聤耳方。

末石硫黃，以粉耳中，日一夜一。

治小兒耳瘡方。

燒馬骨灰敷之。

又方
燒雞屎白，筒中吹入。

Commentary IX.19.a ⧫ Sabine Wilms

The present translation follows Wiseman's terminological choice for the pathology 聤耳 *tíng ěr*. According to the entry on this condition in vol. 48 of the *Zhū Bìng Yuán Hòu Lùn*, "The ears are the gathering place of the ancestral vessels and the place where kidney qì penetrates. In small children, the kidney *zàng* organ is exuberant. When you then have heat present, the heat qì will rise and surge into the ears, the fluids will get congested, and hence pus will be produced. This disease can also be caused by bathing, if water enters the ears and is not fully drained out by tilting the ears. As a result, water damp collects and strikes the blood and qì. Binding with warmth, it produces heat, which also causes the discharge of pus. Both of these etiologies can cause purulent ears. If it is not cured for a long time, it transforms and produces deafness."

IX.19 Ear Problems

IX.19.a Formula for Purulent Ears

Indication
A formula for small children, to treat purulent ears.

Ingredients and Preparation
Pulverize *shíliúhuáng* and sprinkle it into the ears, once during the day and once at night.

IX.19.b Formulas for Ear Sores

Unnamed Formula
Indication
A formula for small children to treat ear sores.

Ingredients and Preparation
Char horse bones into ashes and spread [on the sores].

Another Formula
Char white chicken manure and blow it into the ear by means of a bamboo tube.

衍義

（一）硫黃溫散，專治陰中蘊積之垢。

（二）馬骨灰袪風散熱。

（三）雞屎白下氣散濕。

（四）審其因而用之。

Treatments for Ear Problems *Yăn Yì* (Expanded Meaning)

(1) *Shíliúhuáng* is warm and dissipating and specifically treats filth that is smoldering and collecting within yīn.

(2) Ashes from [charred] horse bones expel wind and dissipate heat.

(3) White chicken manure moves qì down and dissipates dampness.

(4) Use [these formulas] after you have discerned the [specific] cause [of the disease].

Commentary Ear Problems *Yăn Yì* ❧ Sabine Wilms

陰中 *yīn zhōng*: I have purposely left this phrase in a literal translation so that readers can make up their own mind on how to interpret this phrase. "Within yīn" could mean "inside locations that are yīn by nature," i.e., places that are shady, internal, damp, cool etc. In that case, the ear canal would be only one of many possible locations for which *Shíliúhuáng* is indicated. Alternatively, the phrase could refer to the kidney as the most yīn of all organs and the deepest layer of yīn in the body, of which the ears are merely the outside manifestation. It is up to you, the reader, how specific or broad you want to read the meaning of "yīn" in this specific context.

治小兒齒落，久不生方。

以牛屎中大豆二七枚，小開豆頭以注齒根處，數度即生。

又方

（一）取雄鼠屎三七枚，以一屎拭一齒根處，盡此止，二十一日即生。

（二）雄鼠屎頭尖。

IX.20 Tooth Problems

Unnamed Formula

Indications

A formula for small children, to treat loss of teeth without forming new ones for a long time.

Ingredients and Preparation

Take two times seven large beans from inside cow manure,
slightly open the tip of the beans and pour [the liquid emerg-
ing from there?][58] on the location of the roots of the teeth. After
doing this several times, [the new teeth] will form.

Another Formula

(1) Take three times seven droppings from a male mouse and
rub each dropping on the location of one tooth's root. Stop
when you have used up all [the droppings]. After twen-
ty-one days, [the new teeth] will form.

(2) The droppings from male mice are pointed at the tip.

---

58 Researching the composition of cow manure in early medieval China to
determine the identity of these "large beans" unfortunately falls outside the
framework of this book. Presumably it would depend on cattle grazing patterns, the seasonal cycle, and agricultural crops of any specific area, to name
just a few starting points.

衍義

（一）齒屬腎，而鼠屎專資天一生水之源。

（二）或用砭針出血，以鼠骨灰操揩。尤效。

Treatments for Tooth Problems *Yǎn Yì* (Expanded Meaning)

(1) The teeth are associated with the kidney, and mouse droppings specifically serve as provision for this source of water, which is produced from the Heavenly One. [59]

(2) Alternatively, use a lancing stone or needle and make [the gums] bleed. Hold ashes from [charred] mouse bones and wipe them [across the bleeding gums]. Outstanding efficacy!

---

59 The frequent presence of mouse droppings or charred mouse parts as components of pediatric formulas is striking. The *Běncǎo Gāngmù* does have an entry on mouse as a medicinal ingredient but merely mentions its effect in treating miscarriage and easing childbirth. Moreover, it quotes Táo Hóng-jǐng, among others, as already explaining that "mouse" (鼠 *shǔ*) in the context of materia medica literature actually refers to 鼯鼠 *wú shǔ*, which is a flying squirrel. Its medicinal effects are related to the fact that it is a breastfeeding mammal that is able to fly. By contrast, the use of mouse in the pediatric formulas of the *Qiān Jīn Fāng* seems to be related to its ability to support the newborn child's congenital "Earlier Heaven" endowment of qì. Given its use for treating problems with teeth here and sores in the ears below, it could be related to the fact that the mouse or rat is the animal associated with the earthly branch 子 *zǐ* and as such with yáng water, the winter solstice, the kidney, and the storage function. I am grateful to Lorraine Wilcox for reminding me of this connection.

治小兒四五歲不語方。

末赤小豆，酒和敷舌下。

又
灸足兩踝各三壯。

衍義

（一）赤小豆上通心包，下達小腸，乃清熱利竅
之品。

（二）得酒和傅舌下，滲入廉泉，則心胞清淨，
而聰自發於靈臺，慧自達於喉舌矣。

Commentary IX.21 ☙ Julian Scott

In children who are four or five years of age and show no
other signs of developmental problems, inability to speak
is usually due to a local weakness in the area of the tongue,
as well as weakness in the heart and pericardium channels.

This moxa treatment may be related to the fact that the tip of
the external malleolus treats the jaw and tongue.

IX.21 Inability to Speak

Indication

A formula for small children, to treat failure to speak at the age of four or five *suì*.

Ingredients and Preparation

Pulverize *chìxiǎodòu* and mix with liquor. Apply this to the area below the tongue.

Another [Method]

Treat both ankles of the feet with moxibustion, burning three cones on each on.

Treatments for Inability to Speak *Yǎn Yì* (Expanded Meaning)

(1) *Chìxiǎodòu* moves upward to free the flow to the pericardium and moves downward to reach the small intestine. It is indeed a heat-clearing and orifice-disinhibiting substance.

(2) Combining it with liquor and applying this under the tongue where it percolates into Liánquán causes the pericardium to become clear and pure. As a result, acuity spontaneously springs forth from Língtái[60] while intelligence is spontaneously transmitted to the throat and tongue.

---

60 Literally translated, 靈臺 *líng tái* means "platform of numinosity" (if we must give the difficult character 靈 *líng* an English translation). Originally a name to refer to various architectural structures used by rulers for purposes like astronomical observation, in the context of the human body it has been used to refer to the heart (as in the 庚桑楚 *Gēng Sāng Chǔ* chapter of the *Zhuāngzǐ*) or, in Daoist cultivation literature, to the head. In a more strictly medical sense, it is best known as the name of the acupuncture point known in modern times simply as "GV-10."

治小兒數歲不行方。

取葬家未開戶，盜食來以哺之，日三，便起行。

治小兒不能乳方。

雀屎四枚，末之，著乳頭飲兒，兒大十枚。

衍義

（一）雀屎專滌胃中痰涎垢膩，垢膩清而乳食自
　　　如。

（二）慎勿疑於乳癖，而妄行攻擊也。

IX.22 Inability to Walk

Unnamed Formula
Indication
A formula for small children, to treat inability to walk at the age of several *suì*.

Ingredients and Preparation
Choose a household that has just had a funeral but has not yet opened its doors again, and steal some food from them. Feed this to the child, three times a day. Then he or she will begin to walk.

IX.23 Inability to Nurse

Unnamed Formula
Indication
A formula for small children, to treat inability to nurse.

Ingredients and Preparation
Pulverize four sparrow droppings and make them adhere to the nipple. Have the child drink from there. If the child is older, use ten droppings.

Treatment for Inability to Nurse *Yǎn Yì* (Expanded Meaning)

(1) Sparrow droppings specifically sweep phlegm-drool, filth, and slime out of the stomach. When the filth and slime are cleared, the child will nurse and eat with ease.

(2) Beware that you do not [falsely] suspect milk aggregations and recklessly carry out an attack.

蒲黃湯

治小兒落床墜地，如有瘀血，腹中，陰陰寒熱，
不肯乳哺，但啼哭叫喚方。

蒲黃	各十銖
大黃	
黃芩	
甘草	八銖
麥門冬	十銖
芒硝	七銖
黃連	十二銖

IX.24 Púhuáng Tāng (Typha Pollen Decoction)

Indications

A formula for small children, to treat having fallen off the bed or being dropped to the ground, with an appearance suggesting the presence of static blood, a deep chronic pain inside the abdomen, [alternating] cold and heat, and no interest in nursing or being fed but only crying and wailing.

Ingredients

púhuáng	
dàhuáng	10 *zhū* each
huángqín	
gāncǎo	8 *zhū*
màiméndōng	10 *zhū*
mángxiāo	7 *zhū*
huánglián	12 *zhū*

Commentary IX.24 ❧ Sabine Wilms

According to the *Zhū Bìng Yuán Hòu Lùn*, "The symptom of stasis damage in small children who have fallen off the bed is as follows: Regarding the blood in the body, it moves by following the qì and normally does not have a place where it stops and collects. If the movement of blood has lost its proper measure because of injuries from falling or being dropped, it stops in the location of the injury. If it has streamed into the abdomen, it also gathers there without dispersing and always forms static blood. Whenever static blood is present internally, the facial complexion turns withered yellow, breathing becomes faint and panting, rough and unsmooth with minor cold or buzzing and droning with slight heat, and possibly occasional stabbing pain."

（一）上七味，咬咀，以水二升，煮取一升，去
滓，納芒硝。

（二）分三服，消息視兒，羸瘦半之，大小便血
即愈。忌冷食。

衍義

（一）乳哺啼叫，明系火氣用事；腹中陰陰定屬
血滯有形。

（二）故需蒲黃、芒硝以散瘀積，芩、連、大黃
以瀉胎熱，門冬、甘草以滋胃中津氣。

（三）非審證之確，何能至此。

Preparation

(1) Of the seven ingredients, pound [the herbs] and decoct in 2 *shēng* of water until reduced to 1 *shēng*. Remove the dregs and add the *mángxiāo*.

(2) Divide into three doses. Take your time[61] to observe the child. If [the patient] is markedly emaciated, cut the dosage in half. When there is blood in the patient's urine and feces, this means recovery.[62] Cold foods are contraindicated.

---

61   消息 *xiāo xī*: This term has several meanings that could apply here, giving the line a slightly different meaning. It can simply mean "to take a rest," but also "to deliberate" or even "waxing and waning," "increasing and decreasing." In any case, I read it as a warning to diagnose the situation carefully before taking action, which makes solid clinical sense, given the urgency and danger of misdiagnosing such a precarious situation.

62   At first sight, the detection of blood in the patient's urine or feces might be taken as a reason for alarm. Nevertheless, we must remember that the other symptoms in this condition are the result of blood collecting and staying in the injured location instead of moving freely as it does in a healthy person. As such, the elimination of blood with the urine or feces is a positive sign that the medicine is having the intended effect of dispersing the static blood from the site of the injury.

Treatment of Injuries from Falling or Being Dropped *Yǎn Yì* (Expanded Meaning)

(1) Crying and wailing while nursing or being fed is clearly tied to fire qì being active. A deep chronic pain in the abdomen certainly is associated with blood stagnation that is assuming a solid shape.

(2) Therefore *púhuáng* and *mángxiāo* are needed to dissipate stasis accumulations; *huángqín*, *huánglián* and *dàhuáng* to drain fetal heat; and *màiméndōng* and *gāncǎo* to enrich the fluids and qì in the stomach.

(3) Without discerning the accuracy of these symptoms, how could you arrive at this [conclusion]?

治小兒食不知飢飽方。

鼠屎二七枚，燒為末，服之。

衍義
鼠屎燒灰，以清理先天之虛氣。

IX.25 Lacking a Sense of Hunger or Satiety

Unnamed Formula

Indication

A formula for small children, to treat lacking a sense of hunger or satiety when eating.

Ingredients and Preparation

Char two times seven mouse droppings and pulverize them. Have the patient ingest this.

> ### *Yǎn Yì* (Expanded Meaning)
>
> Mouse droppings charred into ashes are used to clear and structure the vacuous qì of Earlier Heaven.

治小兒食土方。

取肉一斤，繩系曳地行數里，勿洗，火炙與吃之。

衍義

取血肉之物，沾行動之土，炙而食之，以攻中土蟲積，投其所喜，以誘入蟲口也。

IX.26 Eating Dirt

Unnamed Formula

Indication

A formula for small children, to treat eating dirt.

Ingredients and Preparation

Take 1 *jīn* of meat, tie a rope to it, and drag it over the ground, walking several miles. Do not wash it! Roast it over the fire and have the patient eat it.

Treatment for Eating Dirt *Yǎn Yì* (Expanded Meaning)

We take an object of flesh and blood, get it stained by dirt that people have walked on, then roast it and make the patient eat it. This is done to attack the worm accumulations in the center in earth [of the five phases]. Feeding [the worms] what they like is meant to lure [the medicine] into the worms' mouth.[63]

63 My best guess is that this means that you are feeding the worms flesh and blood, which is what they love to eat, as a lure to get them to consume the medicinal substance, namely the dirt that people have walked on.

治小兒噦方。

生薑汁	各五合
牛乳	

上二味，煎取五合，分為二服。

又方

取牛乳一升，煎取五合，分五服。

衍義

（一）噦屬胃氣虛寒，牛乳滋胃中血氣，薑汁散胃中虛冷。

（二）亦素禀多火，火逆上沖而噦，但取牛乳潤燥，不得複用薑汁。

IX.27 Vomiting

Indication
A formula for small children, to treat vomiting.

Ingredients

fresh ginger juice	5 gě each
cow's milk	

Preparation
Take the two ingredients above and decoct until reduced to 5 gě. Divide into two doses.

Another Formula
Take 1 shēng of cow's milk and decoct it until reduced to 5 gě. Divide into five doses.

Treatments for Vomiting Yǎn Yì (Expanded Meaning)

(1) Vomiting is associated with vacuity cold in the stomach qì. Cow's milk enriches the blood and qì in the stomach, while ginger juice dissipates vacuity cold inside the stomach.

(2) It is also [possible that the patient is suffering from] a congenital excess of fire, which ascends counterflow and causes the vomiting. Then we only take cow's milk to moisten dryness, but must not also use ginger juice.

治小兒疰方。

灶中灰鹽等分，相和，熬熨之。

衍義

灰鹽溫熨，經脈漸通。

Commentary IX.28 ◂ Sabine Wilms

疰 *Zhù* refers to conditions that are characterized by infections that become chronically lodged (such as summer infixation, 疰 夏 *zhù xià*, or worm infixation, 疰蟲 *zhù chóng*). It is often used interchangeably with 注 *zhù* ("influx") but also carries the connotation of 住 *zhù* ("to stay") based on their related etymology. In its narrowest and most serious sense as "corpse influx" (尸注 *shī zhù*), *zhù* (whether written as 注 or as 疰) is described in the *Zhū Bìng Yuán Hòu Lùn* as a dreadful condition caused by externally contracted ghost evil, which leads to increasing suffering from intermittent cold and heat, urinary problems, general severe discomfort, confusion, panting, and pain in the abdomen, heart, rib-side, lumbus, and back. Eventually it results in death. Being highly contagious after death, it is likely to be passed on to other members of the family (《病源論》 23:2:6). See also Wiseman and Féng, *Practical Dictionary*, p. 300, and 《中華醫學大辭典》 p. 1087. For a detailed analysis of 疰 by medieval medical writers, see Michel Strickman, *Chinese Magical Medicine*, pp. 23-34. See *Zhū Bìng Yuán Hòu Lùn* vol. 47 on 注 *zhù* in the context of pediatrics, and vol. 24 on the "various types of infixation" 諸疰 *zhū zhù*.

IX.28 Infixation

Indication

A formula for small children, to treat infixation.

Ingredients and Preparation

Take equal amounts of stove ash and salt and mix them well. Toast this mixture and apply as a hot compress.

Treatment for Infixation *Yǎn Yì* (Expanded Meaning)

When ashes and salt are applied as a warm compress, the flow in the channels and vessels is gradually opened up again.

治小兒誤吞針方。

取磁石如棗核大，吞之及含之，其針立出。

治小兒誤吞鐵等物方。

艾蒿一把，剉，以水五升，煮取一升半，服之即下。

IX.29 Retrieving Swallowed Objects

IX.29.a Retrieving a Swallowed Needle

Indication
A formula for small children, to treat accidental swallowing of a needle.

Ingredients and Preparation
Take a magnet the size of a jujube pit and swallow it or hold it in the mouth. The needle will emerge immediately.

IX.29.b Retrieving Swallowed Metal Objects

Indication
A formula for small children, to treat accidentally swallowing iron or similar substances.

Ingredients and Preparation
Take a handful of *àihāo* and chop it. Decoct it in 5 *shēng* of water until reduced to 1.5 *shēng*. Having the patient ingest this will move [the object] down.[64]

---

64   The intended action of this formula is thus to have the stuck object move down through the digestive tract and eventually out of the body by means of defecation.

衍義

（一）磁石引針，如母召子，含則取其上引，吞
可使隨下脫。

（二）艾蒿下鐵，取其純陽以運重著。

（三）何憚不下趨耶。

治小兒蠷螋咬，繞腹匝即死方。

（一）搗蒺藜葉敷之。

（二）無葉，子亦可。

又方

取燕窠中土，豬脂和敷之，乾則易之。

Retrieving Swallowed Objects *Yǎn Yì* (Expanded Meaning)

(1) A magnet draws the needle to it like a mother calling a child to her side. When holding [the magnet] in the mouth, this method takes advantage of its ability to draw [the object] upward. Swallowing it allows [the patient] to get rid of [the object] by making it follow [the magnet] downward.

(2) *Àihāo* moves the iron downward, taking advantage of its pure yáng nature to move heavy objects.

(3) Why would you fear that you cannot rush [things] down [and out of the body]!

IX.30 Earwig Bites

Indication
A formula for small children, to treat earwig bites that result in death if the [infection] encircles the abdomen.

Ingredients and Preparation
(1) Pound *jílí* leaves and spread them on [the bite].

(2) If you do not have leaves, you can also use the seeds.

Another Formula
Take dirt from inside a swallow's nest and mix it with lard. Spread this on [the bites] and change it when it has dried.

衍義

（一）蠼螋稟陰濕毒，故其溲著人皮膚，即時腐
爛。

（二）《千金》取白蒺藜葉傳之，以其能散惡血
也。

（三）胡燕窠中土，豬脂和傳，以其能收濕解毒
也。

（四）近世以鐵鏽水除蠼螋瘡，取其墜熱開結，
平肝消腫也。

（五）張介賓曰：《千金》小兒諸證，無所不備，
獨不及痘疹之方者，以痘疹起於南粵，斯
時秦中尚無此患耳。

Treatments for Earwig Bites *Yǎn Yí* (Expanded Meaning)

(1) Earwigs are endowed with the toxicity of yīn dampness. Therefore when their urine comes into contact with a person's skin, it immediately causes putrefaction.

(2) The reason why the *Qiān Jīn Fāng* chooses white *jílí* leaves to apply to [the bite] is that they are able to dissipate malign blood.

(3) The rationale for applying dirt from inside a swallow's nest mixed with lard to [the bites] is that it is able to astringe dampness and resolve toxin.

(4) In modern times, people use rust water to eliminate earwig sores, taking advantage of its ability to weigh down heat and open binds, calm the liver and disperse swelling.

(5) A quote from Zhāng Jièbīn: Among all the disease patterns for small children, there are none that the *Qiān Jīn Fāng* does not provide treatments for. The reason why the text only fails to include formulas for smallpox is that smallpox began in the South. In [Sūn Sīmiǎo's] times, this disease did not yet exist in the area of Qín.[65]

---

65 秦 Qín: This is the historical name given to the region where Sūn Sīmiǎo lived, in modern-day Shǎnxī Province.

Weights and Measures

Weights

1 *shǔ* 黍	=	millet grain
1 *zhū* 銖	=	10 *shǔ* 黍
1 *fēn* 分	=	6 *zhū* 銖
1 *liǎng* 兩	=	24 *zhū* 銖
1 *jīn* 斤	=	16 *liǎng* 兩

Volume

1 *dāo guī* 刀圭	=	4 *wú tóng* 梧桐
1 *cuō* 撮	=	4 *dāo guī* 刀圭
1 *sháo* 勺	=	10 *cuō* 撮
1 *gě* 合	=	2 *sháo* 勺
1 *shéng* 升	=	10 *gě* 合
1 *dǒu* 斗	=	10 *shéng* 升
1 *hú* 斛		10 *dǒu* 斗

Length

1 *cùn* 寸	=	10 *fēn* 分
1 *chǐ* 尺	=	10 *cùn* 寸
1 *bù* 步	=	5 *chǐ* 尺
1 *lǐ* 里	=	1800 *chǐ* 尺

Single Herb & Formula Index

J

K

L

M

N

P

Q

Y

Z

Indications Index

hands, 57, 179, 285, 297
hardness and tension in the heart and abdomen, 39
headache, 147
heat
  abiding heat [that was contracted] in utero, 157
  fetal heat, 361, 485
  fulminant presence of heat, 33
  generalized heat, 5, 27, 35, 39, 147, 175, 247
  heat effusion, 5, 25, 27, 71, 163, 173, 175, 189, 199, 377, 421, 426
  heat in the head and face, 11
  presence of heat without sweating, 79
  severe generalized heat, 35
  tidal heat, 49, 51
  vexing heat, 61, 85, 179
  vigorous heat, 55, 59, 63, 65, 173, 189, 377, 421
  wind heat, 9, 237, 241, 263, 267, 281, 343, 349, 375, 417, 437, 447
heavy inhaling in the chest, 107
hematuria, 447, 451
hypertonicity, 157, 291, 293, 397

I

inability to be at ease, 137
inability to eat and drink, 177, 426
inability to nurse, 481
inability to walk, 387, 481
inch whiteworm, 441
infixation, 492-493
inhibited breathing, 57
inhibition in the triple burner, 53
inhibited defecation and urination, 39, 147
intrusive upset, 173
itch, 237, 267, 285, 289, 291, 299
itching, 271, 285, 297, 311, 408, 411

wind itch, 285, 289, 291

J

jaundice, 75, 77, 157

L

lack of appetite, 109, 163, 195
lack of attunement in the qì of the stomach, 195
lacking a sense of hunger, 487
leprosy, 267, 271, 281, 285
loss of teeth, 475
lusterless skin, 285

M

macules, 3, 7
malaria, 51, 85, 87
malign, 137, 139, 225, 237, 251, 281, 287, 305, 309, 315, 327, 337, 361, 367, 375, 394-395, 499
malignity strike, 173
mild swelling, 57
mouth
  malign sores on the sides of the mouth, 367
  Yellow Flesh and Sores on the Bottom of the Mouth, 367

N

nasal congestion, 97, 285, 465, 467
nasal and oral discharge, 107
navel, 261, 335-337, 339, 341, 343, 391, 425, 451
  incessant oozing, 341
  not healing, 423
  red and swollen navel, 341
  wind navel, 336-337
neck, 236, 243, 377
nodes, 236-237, 243, 245, 421
nose, 75, 77, 323, 428, 465, 469

wind strike, 371
wind toxin, 245, 249, 287, 305,
    329, 361, 375, 395
worms, 81, 279, 283, 305, 327, 331,
    408, 426-428, 432-433, 437, 443,
    445, 489

Proper Name Index

T

W

X

Y

Z

General Index

A

Abate, 41
 Abates, 45
 Abating, 43, 73
Abduct, 261
 Abducts, 375, 383
Abiding, 43, 47, 109, 157, 159, 161, 163, 177, 189
Abscesses, 229
Absence, 463
Absentmindedness, 432
Accumulate, 7, 99, 129, 201
 Accumulating, 69, 146, 184, 405
Accumulation, 164, 423, 429
 Accumulations, 98, 181, 185, 189, 425, 453, 485, 489
Acorus, 129, 131
Acrid, 13, 33, 131, 155, 157, 159, 185, 225
Acridity, 119, 127
Acuity, 479
Adult, 109, 309
Advances, 45
 Advancing, 43, 71
Advice, 226
Advised, 31
Affect, 317
 Affected, 257, 259, 263, 283, 293
 Affecting, 377, 433
 Affects, 407
Affliction, 267
Agent, 336
Ages, 187
Aggravated, 103
Aggressively, 90
Alter, 51
Alternating, 163-164, 483
Alternatingly, 271
Alternative, 71, 101

Alum, 211
Anal, 423, 425
Ancestral, 397, 470
Anesthetics, 206
Angelica, 207
Anger, 397
Angry, 237, 452
Animal, 226
Anise, 23, 25
Ankle, 357
 Ankles, 479
Ankyloglossia, 351
Anterior, 385
Antibiotics, 99, 206, 269
Appear, 94, 317, 396, 408
Appearance, 109, 385, 396, 483
Appearing, 433
Appetite, 109, 146, 163-164, 195, 428
Apricot, 117, 119, 371
Armpit, 236
Army, 95
Arouse, 63, 189, 453
Ascend, 390
 Ascended, 193
 Ascends, 491
Ascent, 97, 101, 117, 119, 131, 137
Ash, 225, 327, 408, 493
 Ashed, 327, 329, 375
Aster, 97, 99
Asthma, 137
Astringe, 113, 201, 305, 329, 375, 425, 499
 Astringes, 291, 329, 343
 Astringing, 437
Attack, 67, 87, 327, 331, 481, 489
 Attacking, 189
 Attacks, 25, 213, 343

519